THE
HIGHLY SELECTIVE
DICTIONARY
OF
GOLDEN
ADJECTIVES
FOR THE
EXTRAORDINARILY
LITERATE

Also by Eugene Ehrlich

THE HIGHLY SELECTIVE THESAURUS
FOR THE EXTRAORDINARILY LITERATE

THE HIGHLY SELECTIVE DICTIONARY
FOR THE EXTRAORDINARILY LITERATE

AMO, AMAS, AMAT AND MORE

VENI, VIDI, VICI

LES BON MOTS

THE INTERNATIONAL THESAURUS OF QUOTATIONS
(WITH MARSHALL DEBRUHL)

THE HARPER DICTIONARY OF FOREIGN TERMS, 3RD EDITION

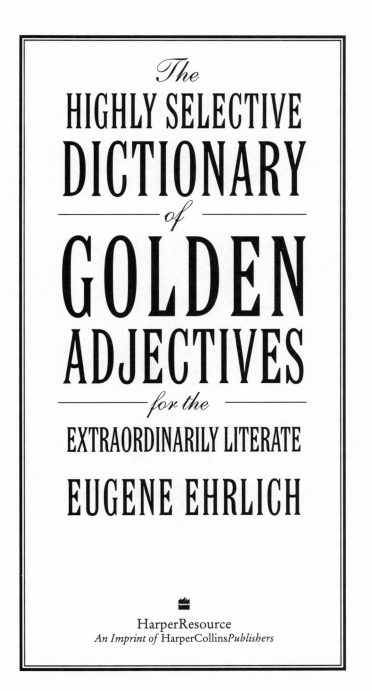

The
HIGHLY SELECTIVE
DICTIONARY
of
GOLDEN
ADJECTIVES
for the
EXTRAORDINARILY LITERATE

EUGENE EHRLICH

HarperResource
An Imprint of HarperCollins*Publishers*

HarperCollins books may be purchased for educational, business, or sales promo-
tional use. For information please write: Special Markets Department, Harper-
Collins Publishers Inc., 10 East 53rd Street, New York, NY 10022.

FIRST EDITION

Library of Congress Cataloging-in-Publication Data has been applied for.

ISBN 0-06-018636-4

02   03   04   05   06   WBC/RRD   10   9   8   7   6   5   4   3   2   1

CONTENTS

ACKNOWLEDGMENTS

To beloved Norma, my wife and most able and discerning reader, whose gift for explication and a keen eye have contributed so much to this book.

To Jason Ehrlich, and to Susan Baxter, who never gives up.

To our four talented children, to Dr. Dan Costin, to our friends Cynthia and Davis Crippen, and to the late Julian Pace and to his wife Dorothy Pace, all of whom helped Norma and me through trying times.

In memory of Daniel and Eileen Murphy, the most faithful of friends.

PREFACE

Something there is in the hearts of teachers and critics of English that finds adjectives the most detestable elements of the language and the most easily excised. Yet, even a brief examination of some of the headwords in the dictionary before you suggests the magnificence of more or less useful English words that are classified as adjectives and enable you to exploit the richness of tone and shades of meaning awaiting your readers.

Consider, for example, what you and other writers would do without the likes of **adventitious** and **aleatory**, **baleful** and **banausic**, **contumelious** and **cunctative**, **diaphanous** and **disingenuous**, **ebullient** and **edacious**, **factitious** and **fatidic**, **gestic** and **gnathonic**, **halcyon** and **heuristic**, **iatrogenic** and **impuissant**, **jejune** and **jocund**, **kempt** and **knurled**, **lambent** and **Laodicean**, **magniloquent** and **marmoreal**, **nescient** and **niveous**, **obdurate** and **officious**, **Panglossian** and **Paphian**, **quaquaversal** and **quixotic**, **redolent** and **refulgent**, **sacerdotal** and **Sisyphean**, **temerarious** and **truculent**, **ulotrichous** and **umbrageous**, **verecund** and **veridical**, **waspish** and **willful**, and **xylophagous**, **yeasty**, and **zaftig**. And these, of course, are just some of the golden adjectives you will meet in this book.

Adjectives have long had bad press in some quarters, and I believe the fault lies with traditional teachers of English. Read on.

Many years have passed since I first teamed up with my colleague Daniel Murphy to write various volumes on grammar and language. In both these disciplines he and I were encouraged to reveal our knowledge and skills to readers as well as to our students. Dan was at Baruch College of the City University and I was at the School of General Studies at Columbia University.

At that time, pompous English teachers were fond of telling their callow students, "Adjectives are the enemy of nouns, and adverbs are the enemy of everything else." I had of course heard this maxim before and believed it without question.

But why did Murphy and I support the advice of such grand announcements? Because we belonged to the generation that recognized Ernest Hemingway as supreme novelistic authority. Ours was the generation in which every English teacher worth his deprived prose was telling students wholesale that Hemingway wrote sentences made up solely of nouns and verbs. Modifiers of any stripe were forbidden. The resulting student sentences turned out to be starved of punctuation and severely sparing of word pictures of action, appearance, aspiration, and feeling— some of the very functions adjectives fulfill especially well.

Having absorbed this attitude from our teachers, we advanced it among our own students. And the pity to this day is that many of today's romantic—even impossibly jaded—teachers of writing persist in giving their students the same incorrect come-on: Want to be Hemingway redivivus? Eschew modifiers.

Readers long have been interested in the strength of the English language and its usefulness in characterizing our aspirations, achievements, and anxieties. Think of those expressions including the adjective "golden." Consider the golden mean, golden handshake, golden bowl, golden wedding, golden fleece, golden age, among many golden others. Then we have such less than glorious expressions as goldbrick, fool's gold, and the golden calf. All with a distinctive charm, and all gold or golden.

The Highly Selective Dictionary of Golden Adjectives for the Extraordinarily Literate offers a compendium of noun modifiers that are golden in the sense of being "brilliant, exceptionally valuable, advantageous, or fine," as suggested in the expression *golden opportunity* or in the title of Lewis Mumford's wonderful literary study *The Golden Day*. Can there be anything better than golden?

In this vein, *The Highly Selective Dictionary* was conceived as a highly personal tribute to the most interesting of the words awaiting you to help adorn, sharpen, and amplify your English sentences. For this is what adjectives are intended to do. And golden adjectives do this better than most. How could they not?

The Highly Selective Dictionary is certainly not a *permissive* dictionary. Permissive dictionaries are excessively tolerant and inclusive of any words or any spellings that come along. And if people don't know what a word means or how it is spelled, such dictionaries make an educated guess, no matter how misleading.

In contrast, The Highly Selective Dictionary is a *prescriptive* dictionary, one whose ultimate task is to reward deserving words with inclusion if they have exhibited plentiful signs of being and remaining useful in our language. The *prescriptive* editor attempts to define and spell these words carefully and conservatively, trying always to tell readers what the selected words usually mean and how they are most often spelled, and not settle for what an editor thinks readers may some day believe those words mean.

I consider myself privileged to have selected this list of English adjectives—not the entire list of adjectives known to exist, of course, but those golden adjectives I consider to be of greatest interest and possible usefulness for readers, writers, and students. This chance to write about adjectives provides a third volume of parallel works concerning our language, which begin with *The Highly Selective Thesaurus for the Extraordinarily Literate* and continue with *The Highly Selective Dictionary for the Extraordinarily Literate*, both also published by HarperCollins.

My hope is that readers will find these golden adjectives useful and entertaining. Thus, each entry begins with an adjectival headword and its pronunciation, and goes on to offer etymological information, definitions, and examples of usage. Finally, words related in meaning to the headwords are supplied, classified, and pronounced.

Eugene Ehrlich
April 4, 2002

PRONUNCIATION NOTES

American pronunciation follows few hard-and-fast rules but may vary from region to region. In pronouncing the headwords of this dictionary, I have considered all the pronunciations given in standard sources and then tried to select the most common ones. Even so, some of the pronunciations supplied inevitably indulge the editor's preferences.

Be advised that in almost every case only one pronunciation is given for a headword, even though some words commonly have multiple pronunciations. You will find that you cannot go wrong with the single pronunciations given. They are always among the correct pronunciations given for these words in unabridged dictionaries.

The respelling pronunciation scheme used is almost identical with the scheme devised for use in my previous *Highly Selective* books and is just as easy to use. Each pronunciation is shown in parentheses just after the headword, and every headword is an adjective, so I have been relieved of the task of telling you ad nauseam that the headwords all are adjectives.

Fully stressed syllables are shown in CAPITAL LETTERS.

Syllables that receive secondary stress are shown in SMALL CAPITAL LETTERS.

Unstressed syllables are shown in lowercase letters, as are pronunciations of words of one syllable.

Here are three examples of pronounced adjectives:

baleful (BAYL-fəl)
unkempt (un-KEMPT)
knurled (nurld)

An exception to respelling is use of the schwa (ə), which is defined as an indistinct or unaccented vowel sound, as in the second syllable of baleful (BAYL-fəl) and the final syllable of ebullient (i-BUUL-yənt). Such pronunciations, involving use of the schwa, occur only in unaccented syllables.

But there are times when not even a schwa is appropriate. This happens when an "l" or "n" is used alone—whispered, really—to pronounce a word, or is used in combination with another consonant and can serve as a syllable without having an accompanying vowel. Consider the word addlepated, which in this book is pronounced (AD-l-PAY-tid). The "l" stands alone without even the help of the schwa, for it does not have the sound of an "l" preceded by a vowel. Consider also the word centripetal, which is pronounced (sen-TRIP-i-tl), and the word fictile (FIK-tl). No schwas are needed. Then there are words pronounced with a single "n," as in glutton (GLUT-n) and in gluttony (GLUT-n-ee), or an "n" linked with a "t," as in wanton (WON-tn) and in succedent (sək-SEED-nt).

Another exception to respelling is the use of ī, ɪ, and Ī to indicate long vowel sounds, as in the first syllable of didactic (dī-DAK-tik) and the second syllable of derisive (di-RĪ-siv). The symbol ɪ indicates the sound of a syllable with secondary stress, but retaining the long vowel sound, as in the third syllable of dewy-eyed, here pronounced DOO-ee-ɪD.

There are two other exceptions to respelling:

The italicized "*th*" is used to show the initial sound of words such as "this" and "thus," which are given as (*th*is) and (*th*us). By contrast, in "thin" and "both," the sound of th is not italicized. An actual adjective in the text is blithesome, pronounced (BLĪ*TH*-səm).

Please note that in the chart that follows, *n* indicates an n that is only partially pronounced, as in many words of French origin.

PRONUNCIATION KEY

a *as in* act, hat, carry
ah *as in* balm, calm, father
ahr *as in* far, jar, darling

air *as in* fairy, scare, declare
aw *as in* audit, walk, gawk, saw
ay *as in* age, bay, heinous
b *as in* bake, babble, boob
ch *as in* choose, church, preach
d *as in* dare, fuddled, mud
e *as in* empty, led, berry
ee *as in* ease, either, meat, see
eer *as in* ear, eerie, pier, sneer
f *as in* fin, daffy, belief
g *as in* gust, bargain, hog
h *as in* hairy, hot, huddle
hw *as in* where, whet, anywhere
i *as in* in, hit, women
ī *as in* bite, light, pie, spy
ī̄ *as in* colonize, sympathize
Ī *as in* mighty, lightning, surprise
j *as in* gin, just, judge, garbage
k *as in* kerchief, spoken, rack
l *as in* lag, ladle, sell
m *as in* many, common, madam
n *as in* note, knee, manner, napkin
n *as in* dénouement, frisson, soupçon
ng *as in* hunger, swinging, bring
o *as in* opportune, hot, crop
oh *as in* oppose, most, toast, sew
oo *as in* oodles, pool, ruler
oor *as in* poor, tour, sure
or *as in* aural, border, mortal
ow *as in* owl, oust, house, allow
oy *as in* oil, join, boy
p *as in* print, paper, sleep
r *as in* rash, tarry, poor
s *as in* cent, scent, lease, lessen
sh *as in* sugar, shush, cash

t *as in* talk, utter, heat
th *as in* think, wrath, loath
th as in then, bother, loathe
u *as in* ugly, mutter, come
ur *as in* urge, her, fir, saboteur
uu *as in* brook, full, woman
v *as in* very, every, brave
w *as in* well, awash, allow
y *as in* yet, abeyance, useful
z *as in* zap, gazebo, tease
zh *as in* pleasure, vision, persiflage

Note: Headwords that are considered still to be foreign terms are given in italics.

Note further: No mention is made in this book of the word "entrepreneur" or its adjectival form, in hope that one day presidents and CEOs will all be able to say AHN-trə-prə-NUR or something like it instead of enforcing a rhyme with "sewer."

A

abashed (ə-BASHT)
From Middle English *abaishen*, meaning "to bring low, put down."

1. ashamed or embarrassed.

"A major-league second baseman cannot help feeling **abashed** when he finds himself unable to throw accurately to first base."

2. disconcerted.

"The boy was thoroughly **abashed** when, for the first time in his life, he faced having to use three forks to eat dinner and had no idea which to employ first."

Related words: **abash** (ə-BASH) *verb*; **abashedly** (ə-BASH-id-lee) *adverb*; **abashedness** (ə-BASH-id-nis) and **abashment** (ə-BASH-mənt) *both nouns.*

abdominous (ab-DOM-ə-nəs)
From Latin *abdomen*, meaning "paunch, belly; gluttony."

1. potbellied.

"The tailor made a rich living through his specialty of accommodating comfortably **abdominous** clients who knew he would do everything possible to obscure their overeating."

2. having a paunch or prominent belly.

"The shah's collection of uncorseted, **abdominous** wives may not have appealed to Westerners, but it made him the envy of lecherous old men in his court."

Related words: **abdomen** (AB-də-mən) *noun*; **abdominal** (ab-DOM-ə-nl) *adjective*; **abdominally** (ab-DOM-i-nə-lee) *adverb*.

aberrant (ə-BER-ənt)

From Latin *aberrans*, present participle of verb *aberrare*, meaning "to wander."

1. straying from an expected course, for example, a moral standard.

"In the interest of preserving impeccable reputations, even the youngest divinity students eschewed **aberrant** behavior of any kind."

2. exceptional; deviating widely from the normal type; abnormal; irregular.

"School psychologists today are challenged to distinguish between adolescent experimentation and seriously **aberrant** behavior."

Related words: **aberration** (AB-ə-RAY-shən), **aberrance** (ə-BER-əns), and **aberrancy** (ə-BER-ən-see) *all nouns*; **aberrantly** (ə-BER-ənt-lee) *adverb*.

abortifacient (ə-BOR-tə-FAY-shənt)

From Latin *aboriri*, meaning "to miscarry"; past participle *abortus*. The word is used as a noun in such sentences as "The young pharmacist still blushed slightly after dispensing prescribed **abortifacients**."

causing abortion.

Abortifacient pills have recently been approved for distribution in the United States for termination of early pregnancies."

Related words: **abortive** (ə-BOR-tiv) *adjective*; **abortively** (ə-BOR-tiv-lee) *adverb*; **abortiveness** (ə-BOR-tiv-nis) and **abortus** (ə-BOR-təs) *both nouns*.

abstergent (ab-STUR-jənt)

From Latin *abstergere*, meaning "to wipe off"; present participle *abstergens*.

cleansing, scouring.

"We recognized that at least two applications of an **abstergent** substance would be needed if we were to prepare the fuselage skin properly for space travel."

Abstergent is also used as a noun in such sentences as "Application of even copious amounts of the recommended **abstergent** has no effect on the stain."

Related words: **abstersive** (ab-STUR-siv) *adjective*; **abstersiveness** (ab-STUR-siv-nis) *noun*.

abysmal. *See* **abyssal.**

abyssal (ə-BIS-əl)

From Late Latin adjective *abyssalis*, meaning "of an abyss, of the bowels of the earth."

Abyss as a noun is much more common than the adjective and is used literally and figuratively: "Father Blair's homily never left any doubt he was talking of the gap between parents and their adolescent children, when he spoke of 'the great **abyss.**'"

immeasurable; unfathomable; bottomless; literally pertaining to great ocean depths, for example, between 13,000 and 21,000 feet.

"The depth of his misunderstanding of physics was **abyssal,** and there was no quick way he could overcome it."

"Although the first deep-sea divers expanded **abyssal** knowledge, the natural fears of crew members severely limited their further explorations."

Related words: **abysmal** (ə-BIZ-məl) *adjective*; **abyss** (ə-BIS) and **abysm** (ə-BIZ-əm) *both nouns*.

adamant. *See* **adamantine.**

adamantine (AD-ə-MAN-teen)

From Latin adjective *adamantinus*, meaning "adamantine"; from noun *adamas*, meaning "hard metal; diamond."

Far more common in English is the adjective **adamant,** meaning "unshakable; inflexible," as in "For reasons never explained, the department head remained **adamant** in refusing the annual award to beautiful young women."

immovable; unyielding; obdurate; too hard to pierce or break.

"**Adamantine** in his refusal to compromise his mission, willing to suffer any threatened torture, the young captain firmly stood his ground."

"When all their efforts failed in their attempt to cut the **adamantine** stone, they were finally convinced they had found a potentially valuable diamond."

Related words: **adamant** (AD-ə-mənt) *adjective*; **adamantly** (AD-ə-mənt-lee) *adverb*; **adamance** (AD-ə-məns) and **adamancy** (AD-ə-mən-see) *both nouns*.

addled and **addlebrained**. *See* **addlepated**.

addlepated (AD-l-PAY-tid)

From Middle English *adel*, meaning "rotten," + *pate*, meaning "head."

Also given as **addlebrained** (AD-l-BRAYND), with the same meaning.

The related adjective **addled** (AD-ld) has the primary meaning of "muddled, mentally confused," as in "Despite all my efforts to think clearly once again, my memory remained **addled** for many months after surgery."

A secondary meaning is "rotten," as in "I avoided the **addled** eggs we were habitually served in the overseas army, preferring instead to go hungry most days."

foolish, silly; mentally confused.

"Physicians only recently have begun to question whether absent-mindedness and other difficulties may characteristically indicate physically disturbed patients rather than charmingly **addlepated** individuals."

adjunct (AJ-ungkt)

From Latin *adjungere*, meaning "to join to"; past participle *adjunctus*.

Adjunct is also used as a noun, thus abbreviating common designations such as adjunct professor to **adjunct**: "Many colleges got by in difficult times by reducing the number of their well-paid, full-time professors and hiring **adjuncts** at low salaries."

associated or joined with another in a dependent or subordinate relationship to it.

"Much to her surprise, she found that **adjunct** professors, like others in **adjunct** positions, were neither invited to meetings nor allowed to vote on matters of departmental policy."

Related words: **adjunctive** (ə-JUNGK-tiv) *adjective*; **adjunction** (ə-JUNGK-shən) *noun*.

adroit. *See* **maladroit**.

adscititious. *See* **adventitious**.

adventitious (AD-vən-TISH-əs)

From Latin adjective *adventicius*, meaning "foreign, extraneous; unearned."

Also given as **adscititious** (AD-si-TISH-əs), with the same meanings shown below: "Academic honors for the wealthy, **adscititious** rather than earned, fool no one, not even the recipients."

added from without; not inherent or earned; accidental, by chance.

"The chairman inevitably adorned his opening remarks with **adventitious** compliments about his nominees that explained nothing about why he had selected them."

Related words: **adventitiously** (AD-vən-TISH-əs-lee) *adverb*; **adventitiousness** (AD-vən-TISH-əs-nis) *noun*.

aerobic. *See* **antisudorific.**

agminate (AG-mə-nit)

From Latin *agmen*, meaning "army on a march; troop."

Also given as **agminated** (AG-mə-NAY-tid), with the same meanings as given below.

arranged in a group, aggregated.

"His taste runs to random bunches of **agminate** wildflowers, forgetting that when in bloom there would have to be some consideration given to harmonizing colors in adjacent beds."

agrestal. *See* **agrestic.**

agrestic (ə-GRES-tik)

From Latin *agrestis*, meaning "rustic, wild; belonging to the field."

This English adjective is sometimes given as **agrestal** (ə-GRES-tl), also with the meaning of "rustic; rural."

1. rustic, rural.

"Sally enjoyed the peaceful **agrestic** life as an antidote for the city, where she lived while earning her fortune."

2. unpolished, uncouth.

"In all the years they had been together, she had always been repelled by Stanley's **agrestic** behavior, for example, his boisterous manners while playing poker and drinking beer with his friends."

aleatory (AY-lee-ə-TOR-ee)

From Latin noun *aleator* meaning "gambler; dice player"; adjective *aleatorius* meaning "in gambling."

Also given as **aleatoric** (AY-lee-ə-TOR-ik), meaning "done at random": "All those who blindly throw their money into money-hungry slot machines must believe the **aleatoric** devices will somehow favor them."

1. dependent on chance or luck; random, unpredictable.

"The **aleatory** election of such a boor surely could not have been predicted."

2. in law: dependent on unknown contingencies.

"At the time he was thought foolish for entering into an **aleatory** contract, with his only cargo ship at the mercy of unpredictable storms."

allusive (ə-LOO-siv)

From Latin *alludere*, meaning "to play beside"; past participle *allusus*.

1. referring to something inferred or implied.

"Those of us who really want to discover his true meanings must begin by deciphering each of his many **allusive** representations."

2. abounding in indirect references.

"Joyce's **allusive** literary and philosophical prose in *Finnegans Wake* could not have been foreseen by admirers of his admirable collection of fresh, early poetry in *Chamber Music*."

Related words: **allusively** (ə-LOO-siv-lee) *adverb*; **allusion** (ə-LOO-zhən) and **allusiveness** (ə-LOO-siv-nis) *both nouns*.

alopecic (AL-ə-PEE-sik)

From Latin *alopecia*, meaning "fox mange," a condition known to have caused loss of hair.

The related noun **alopecia** (AL-ə-PEE-shə) means "baldness."

characterized by loss of hair or baldness.

"Ineffective treatments for **alopecic** conditions almost outnumber those for weight reduction."

altricial (al-TRISH-əl)

From Latin *altrix*, feminine of *altor*, meaning "nourisher; foster father."

of a bird or bird species: helpless at birth and requiring assistance by parents for a time.

"**Altricial** eagles are banded early in their first attempts at flight as part of a program to increase the species' chances for survival."

altruistic (AL-troo-IS-tik)

From French adjective *altruiste,* from French noun *altruisme,* roughly meaning "concern for others."

motivated by unselfish concern for the welfare of others.

"Acts of cynical disregard for others cannot easily be counterbalanced by a single **altruistic** deed."

Related words: **altruistically** (AL-troo-IS-ti-kə-lee) *adverb;* **altruism** (AL-troo-IZ-əm) and **altruist** (AL-troo-ist) *both nouns.*

ambagious (am-BAY-jəs)

From French *ambagieux,* from Latin *ambagiosus,* meaning "circuitous, roundabout."

1. circumlocutory, roundabout.

"The old senator's proclivity for **ambagious** oration bored his audience."

2. circuitous, winding; tortuous.

"Does the professor really believe her **ambagious** claptrap can convince any students to abandon their strike?"

Related words: **ambagiousness** (am-BAY-jəs-nis) *noun;* **ambagiously** (am-BAY-jəs-lee) *adverb.*

ambidextrous. *See* **ambisinister.**

ambisinister (AM-bi-SIN-ə-stər) or **ambisinistrous** (AM-bi-SIN-is-trəs).

Both adjectives are from Latin *ambi-,* meaning "both," + Latin *sinister,* meaning "left"; hence, **ambisinister** means "awkward or unfavorable," the opposite of adroit.

The reader would do well to know the adjectival antonym **ambidextrous** (AM-bi-DEK-strəs), which is much more common, and means "able to use both hands equally well." Thus, "When a team has a healthy Bernie Williams ready to hit well from either side of home plate, the value of being **ambidextrous** is readily apparent."

clumsy with both hands.

"Few major league baseball players are truly ambidextrous, but none of them are **ambisinistrous,** because clumsy players rarely get to the major leagues."

Related words: **ambidexterity** (AM-bi-dek-STER-i-tee) and **ambidextrousness** (AM-bi-DEK-strəs-nis) *both nouns;* **ambidextrously** (AM-bi-DEKS-trəs-lee) *adverb.*

amygdaline (ə-MIG-də-lin)

From Latin *amygdalinus*, from Greek *amygdálinos*, both meaning "of almonds."

resembling almonds; related to almonds.

"About all he remembered of the lovely woman were her dark **amygdaline** eyes, which seemed always to have understood everything and offered nothing."

Related words: **amygdaloid** (ə-MIG-də-LOYD), **amygdalate** (ə-MIG-də-lit), **amygdaliform** (ə-MIG-də-lə-FORM), and **amygdalaceous** (ə-MIG-də-LAY-shəs) *all adjectives.*

anaphrodisiac (an-AF-rə-DEE-zee-AK)

From Greek *anaphrodisiakós*, meaning "unable to inspire sexual appetite."

Anaphrodisiac is also used as a noun, as is **anaphrodisia** (an-AF-rə-DEE-zhə).

capable of inducing the diminishing of sexual desire.

"We are led to believe certain cathartics are **anaphrodisiac**, suggesting that a potent laxative can hold back mighty Viagra itself if not the waters of Niagara."

See also **aphrodisiac.**

ancillary (AN-sə-LER-ee)

From Latin *ancilla*, meaning "female servant or slave"; related to the adjective *ancillaris*, "having the status of such a person."

The English noun **ancillary** (plural **ancillaries**) means "a person who works in an ancillary capacity." And an **ancilla** is an accessory or an **adjunct.**

1. subordinate, subsidiary.

"Americans pretend no branch of the federal government is ever **ancillary** to any other, even though we all know this is not always true."

2. assisting; auxiliary.

"When the need arises for cutting expenses, a good executive eliminates **ancillary** personnel before considering reduction of those employees performing essential duties."

Related word: **ancilla** (an-SIL-ə) *noun.*

anguilliform (ang-GWIL-ə-FORM)

From Latin *anguilla,* meaning "eel."

Not to be confused with the adjective **anguine** (ANG-gwin), from Latin *anguinus,* meaning "snakelike"; from *anguis,* meaning "snake."

1. eel-shaped.

"When I catch anything **anguilliform,** I put it into a bucket of water reserved for things I will use as bait; I put fish I will eat into a second bucket."

2. of **anguine,** resembling a snake.

"You knew immediately the man couldn't be trusted; indeed, you wouldn't be surprised if that **anguine** creature suddenly slithered away."

anguine. *See* **anguilliform.**

anserine (AN-sə-RĪN)

From Latin *anserinus,* meaning "pertaining to geese"; from Latin *anser,* "a goose."

The first meaning of **anserine** is so firmly attached to the bird, as in the proverbial "silly goose," that for most people it overpowers the literal meaning.

Also given as **anserous** (AN-sə-rəs).

1. silly; stupid.

"There was considerable doubt whether we would be able to find an **anserine** recruit eager to go on such a dangerous mission."

2. gooselike; resembling a goose.

"What a difference in the reputations of swans and geese—both **anserine** birds—the former graceful and dignified, the latter termed outrageously silly."

anserous. *See* **anserine.**

antepenultimate (AN-tee-pi-NUL-tə-mit)

From Latin *antepaenultimus,* meaning "last but two"; from Latin *ante-* "before" + *paen* "almost" + *ultima* "the last."

Especially in the phrase *syllaba antepaenultima,* meaning "last syllable minus two."

third from the end.

"In the last fifty yards, when the marathon runner realized he could hope for no better than an **antepenultimate** finish, his remaining strength suddenly seemed to disappear."

Related word: **antepenult** (AN-tee-PEE-nult) *noun.*

anteprandial. *See* **prandial** and **preprandial.**

anthropophagous (AN-thrə-POF-ə-gəs)

From Latin *anthropophagus,* from Greek *anthropophagía,* both meaning "man-eating, cannibal."

man-eating, cannibal.

"Unquenchable in their search for ever-greater financial profits, moviemakers have fallen into filming frenzied attacks of **anthropophagous** sharks represented as hungry for a few bites of a luscious nymphet."

Related words: **anthropophagic** (AN-thrə-pə-FAJ-ik) and **anthropophagical** (AN-thrə-pə-FAJ-ik-l) *both adjectives;* **anthropophagously** (AN-thrə-POF-ə-gəs-lee) *adverb;* **anthropophagi** (AN-thrə-POF-ə-jī), **anthropophagite** (AN-thrə-POF-ə-jīt), and **anthropophagy** (AN-thrə-POF-ə-JEE) *all nouns.*

antisudorific (AN-tee-soo-də-RIF-ik)

From Neo-Latin *anti-* "against" + *sudor* "sweat" + *-ific* "causing or operating" — together meaning "operating against sweating."

It is interesting that classical Latin had no word corresponding to the English **antisudorific,** and we had to wait until Neo-Latin invented something close to it, in the adjective *sudorificus,* meaning "inducing sweat." The point of this discussion is that the ancient Romans apparently lacked self-consciousness when it came time to sweat, and modern persons concern themselves obsessively with exercising hard to induce perspiration and therefore lose weight while simultaneously doing everything they can to mask the telltale aroma that identifies persons breaking a sweat.

It is no wonder the adjective aerobic (air-OH-bik) has caught on so thoroughly in past years, even though men and women have a tough time defining it. For the convenience of the reader, the definition is here supplied: "living on oxygen in the air, in other words requiring the presence of oxygen in order to thrive — and sweat."

inhibiting perspiration.

"Men and women, perhaps between the great Ice Ages, appear to have been content to live close together despite their axillary effusions, but when temperatures have been at their highest, city dwellers in particular have resorted to all sorts of creams, lotions, and gaseous entrapments in an effort to exploit the benefits of copious applications of blissfully **antisudorific** substances."

See **axillary.**

aphoristic (AF-ə-RIS-tik)

From the Greek adjective *aphoristikós*, meaning "aphoristic"; from Greek *aphorismós*, meaning "definition; aphorism."

1. containing maxims: short, wise sayings.

   "Professor Barzun seemed to have an endless **aphoristic** trove, and each bon mot he came up with seemed to spawn at least three more, for all of which we were grateful."

2. given to coining maxims.

   "His friends used to label his **aphoristic** penchant 'maximizing' and soon took to calling him 'Max,' a handle short, sweet, and never forgotten."

   Related words: **aphorism** (AF-ə-RIZ-əm), **aphorist** (AF-ər-ist), and **aphorizer** (AF-ə-RĪZ-ər) *all nouns*; **aphorize** (AF-ə-RĪZ) *verb*; **aphoristically** (AF-ə-RIS-ti-klee) *adverb*.

aphrodisiac (AF-rə-DEE-zee-AK)

From Greek *aphrodisiakós*, meaning "relating to love or sex."

Equivalent to Greek *aphrodísios*, meaning "of Aphrodite." Aphrodite, of course, was the ancient Greek goddess of love.

Also given as aphrodisiacal (AF-rə-də-ZĪ-ə-kəl).

arousing sexual desire.

   "He often made a point of dining at expensive Chinese restaurants and always ordered bird's nest soup to exploit its supposed **aphrodisiac** qualities."

   Related word: **aphrodisia** (AF-rə-DEE-zhə) *noun*.

See also **anaphrodisiac.**

apposite (AP-ə-zit)

From Latin *appositus*, meaning "added to, put near"; past participle of *apponere* or *adponere*.

well expressed; appropriate, suitable.

"The best eulogists can expect to be judged only on whether their remarks are **apposite** and brief."

Related words: **appositely** (AP-ə-zit-lee) *adverb*; **appositeness** (AP-ə-zit-nis) and **apposition** (AP-ə-ZISH-ən) *both nouns*.

arena. *See* **arenicolous.**

arenicolous (AR-ə-NIK-ə-ləs)

From Latin *arenicola,* from *arena* "sand" + *cola* "inhabiting." Also given as *harenicola.*

The adjective **arenicolous** should not be confused with **arenose** (AR-ə-NOHS), an adjective meaning "sandy; gritty." Consider the following: "To their surprise, summer residents find that many plants and shrubs can thrive in the **arenose** environments characteristic of seaside homes."

But how does an English word such as "arena" relate to the Latin word *arena,* meaning "sand"? All that is needed to understand this connection is to make a mental jump into an arena of Roman times or even one of modern times. What material usually makes up the floor of the arena? If you answer "sand," the environment is **arenose,** and you win.

inhabiting sand.

"I tried to coax my girlfriend off the hot midday beach by telling her about the horrid habits of **arenicolous** insects living around her, all of which were creatures of my imagination."

Related word: **arenaceous** (AR-ə-NAY-shəs) *adjective.*

arsy-varsy (AHR-see-VAHR-see)

From English **arse** "ass" + Latin *versus* "turned," past participle of *vertere,* "to turn."

A modern version of the colloquial adjective **arsy-varsy** is the equally colloquial "assbackward" or "bassackward," the latter commonly also called a spoonerism. (*See* **bassackwards.**) Bear in mind that the original, vulgar sixteenth-century term may have been *arsey-versy,* but was pronounced in the English of that day as AHR-see-VAHR-see. Hence, today's sensible respelling. So American clerks, not clarks, continue to drink beer, not lager, while watching the Kentucky Derby, not Darby, on television, not the telly.

contrary; perverse, preposterous.

"The boy had an **arsy-varsy** way of complying with his mother's orders that threatened to send the poor woman back to her psychiatrist."

atrabilious (A-trə-BIL-yəs)
From Latin *atra bilis*, meaning "black bile."

The noun *bili* or *bilis*, translated as "bile or gall," is still seen in English in the adjective "bilious," meaning "suffering a surfeit of bile." And **atrabilious** is sometimes given as **atrabiliar** (A-trə-BIL-yər).

But you and I don't concern ourselves with our production of bile. So what does **atrabilious** mean to us? To find out what an excess of black bile can cause, read on, but also see **bilious.**

1. irritable, bad-tempered.

"Trying to navigate a six-lane highway jammed with the same vehicles every day and overcome the road rage he felt left him an **atrabilious** pill-swallower unfit for the day's work he faced."

2. melancholy; gloomy; morose.

"Would you ever believe the breakup of the young man's marriage would leave him an **atrabilious** middle-aged man?"

Related word: **atrabiliousness** (A-trə-BIL-yəs-nis) *noun.*

autochthonous. *See* **heterochthonous.**

avuncular (ə-VUNG-kyə-lər)
From Latin *avunculus*, meaning "maternal uncle"; from Latin *avus*, meaning "grandfather or ancestor."

of or pertaining to a kindly uncle or to someone playing that part.

"If there's anything that all young people find objectionable, it may be the well-meant but insufferable attention given by an **avuncular** relative or friend."

Related words: **avuncularly** (ə-VUNG-kyə-lər-lee) *adverb*; **avuncularity** (ə-vUNG-kyə-LAR-i-tee) *noun.*

axillary (AK-sə-LER-ee)
From Latin *axilla*, meaning "armpit," plural *axillae.*

Also used as a noun in English, **axillar** (AK-sə-lər), meaning "a bird's axillary feather."

pertaining to the human armpit, or to the corresponding underside of a portion of a bird wing.

"A rite of passage for adolescent boys is the inevitable appearance of **axillary** hair, entitling them to smug satisfaction despite having to face a lifetime of exasperatingly dull razors."

B

bacchanal. *See* **bacchanalian.**

bacchanalian (BAK-ə-NAYL-yən)

From Latin *Bacchanalia,* from Greek *Bákhos,* both nouns meaning "a festival in honor of Bacchus," the ancient god of wine.

1. characterized by drunken feasting or by roistering.

   "Try as the students would, their festivities came as close to truly **bacchanalian** intensity as does candle blowing at a child's first birthday party."

2. usually capitalized: relating to a Roman **bacchanal** (BAH-kə-NAHL).

   "What had been supposed to be a wild all-night party turned out to be nothing like the authentic **Bacchanalian** orgy we expected from a department of classical scholars."

   Related words: **Bacchus** (BAK-əs), **Bacchae** (BAK-ee), **bacchante** (bə-KAN-tee), and **bacchanalianism** (BAK-ə-NAYL-yən-iz-əm) *all nouns;* **bacchant** (BAK-ənt) *noun* and *adjective;* **bacchantic** (ba-KAN-tik) and **Bacchic** (BAK-ik) *both adjectives.*

bacciferous. *See* **baccivorous.**

baccivorous. (bak-SIV-ər-əs)

From Latin *bacca,* meaning "berry," + *vorus,* meaning "devouring," together meaning "feeding on berries."

living chiefly on berries.

   "Helen explained that **baccivorous** game birds living in and over brush were much sweeter to eat than birds living on fish."

Related word: **bacciferous** (bak-SIF-ər-əs) *adjective,* meaning producing berries: "Maine's **bacciferous** cranberry vines have established the state as a leading supplier of the unique holiday berries."

balaustine (bə-LAW-stin)

From Latin *balaustium* from Greek *balaústion,* both meaning "pomegranate."

pertaining to the pomegranate.

"Our old-fashioned physician introduced us to poultices made of **balaustine** flowers for treating everyday wounds."

baleful (BAYL-fəl)

From Old English *bealu-full,* meaning "in pain."

pernicious; destructive; noxious.

"His intent was anything but **baleful,** yet he was always considered an outsider in the little town."

Related words: **balefulness** (BAYL-fəl-nis) *noun;* **balefully** (BAYL-fəl-ee) *adverb.*

balneal (BAL-nee-əl)

From Latin *balneum* from Greek *balaneîon,* both meaning "a bath, bathhouse."

pertaining to bathing or baths.

"A seaside town willing to clean its beaches and build bathhouses can create a **balneal** industry that will bring in fresh revenues."

banausic (bə-NAW-sik)

From Greek *banausikós,* meaning "for mechanics."

practical; merely mechanical.

"Frederick claims he is willing to take any kind of job but, when offered an opportunity, describes the work offered as **banausic** and clearly beneath him."

basilic (bə-SIL-ik)

From French *basilique,* from Latin *basilicus,* from Greek *basilikós,* all meaning "royal."

royal, kingly.

"The subjects appeared to stand in awe of her **basilic** majesty, willing to withstand any hardship, face any danger in her behalf."

Related words: **basilican** (bə-SIL-i-kən) and **basilical** (bə-SIL-i-kəl) *both adjectives*; **basilica** (bə-SIL-i-kə) *noun*, meaning a type of church, from Greek *basiliké oikía*, literally "royal house."

The most interesting of related words in this group is a medical term, **basilic vein**, meaning a large vein of great importance located on the inner side of the arm. From Latin *vena basilica*, meaning "royal vein," reminiscent of the Spanish Camino Real, literally "royal road."

bassackwards (BAS-AK-wərdz)

From English slang, popular deliberate spoonerism of **assbackwards**, meaning "in reverse order"; feebly masking the true origin of the word and its supposed vulgarity. Also used as an adverb.

in reverse order.

"My boss frequently gave me the very devil for what he called my daily **bassackwards** routine for organizing the day's work."

benign. *See* **benignant.**

benignant (bi-NIG-nənt)

From the well-known English *benign* + *-ant*, a suffix meaning "characterized by."

1. gracious; kind, especially to inferiors.

"Elizabeth was not admired for her **benignant** manner toward her household servants, whom she considered her inferiors."

2. beneficial; exerting an advantageous influence.

"We were amazed by the immediately **benignant** effect the appointment had on the sagging morale of our company."

Related words: **benign** (bi-NĪN) *adjective*; **benignantly** (bi-NIG-nənt-lee) *adverb*; **benignancy** (bi-NIG-nən-see) *noun*.

bibulous (BIB-yə-ləs)

From Latin *bibulus*, meaning "fond of drink"; from *bibere*, meaning "to drink."

1. fond of alcoholic drink.

"In my undergraduate days I spent many long hours exhibiting my **bibulous** proclivity, so it is no wonder I cannot remember much of what I heard and read in four years at school."

2. spongy; absorbent.

"The **bibulous** cloth seemed to swell to twice its normal size moments after it was dipped in water."

Related words: **bibulously** (BIB-yə-ləs-lee) *adverb*; **bibulousness** (BIB-yə-ləs-nis) and **bibulosity** (BIB-yə-LOS-i-tee) *both nouns.*

bilious (BIL-yəs)

From Latin *biliosus*, meaning "a choleric or bilious man," from *bilis*, meaning "bile or gall, the greenish liquid produced by the liver that assists digestion."

Bile is one of the four principal humors—fluids—in the body: phlegm, blood, choler, and black bile. The predominance of one of these humors in a person was thought to determine the nature of the person's mind and body. Are you phlegmatic, sanguine, choleric, or melancholic?

ill-tempered, peevish, cranky; suffering too great a secretion of bile.

"Newspaper reporters, always under pressure of time and the scrutiny of editors, used to be known for their **bilious** dispositions."

Related words: **biliously** (BIL-yəs-lee) *adverb*; **biliousness** (BIL-yəs-nis) *noun.*

blasé (blah-ZAY)

From French, past participle of *blaser*, meaning "to sicken from excess."

bored with too much of a good thing; bored with excessive worldly pleasures.

"You could tell from the first moment you met him that this was a **blasé** young man who surely would bore or depress all around him."

blasphemous (BLAS-fə-məs)

From Latin *blasphemus* and Greek *blásphemos*, meaning "defaming, speaking evil."

impiously irreverent; profane.

"It was only when the minister began to employ **blasphemous** language in his sermons that we had the first inkling something was seriously affecting him."

Related words: **blasphemously** (BLAS-fə-məs-lee) *adverb*; **blasphemousness** (BLAS-fə-məs-nis), **blasphemy** (BLAS-fə-mee), and **blasphemer** (blas-FEE-mər) *all nouns*; **blaspheme** (blas-FEEM) *verb.*

blithe. *See* **blithesome.**

blithesome (BLĬTH-səm)

From English **blithe** "joyous" + **-some,** a suffix indicating "a quality."

cheerful; merry; lighthearted.

"All of us were sitting together, gloomy about the dangerous operation, but once Alice joined us her **blithesome** spirit lifted our hearts and enabled us to endure."

Related words: **blithe** (blĭth) and **blitheful** (BLĬTH-fəl) *both adjectives;* **blithefully** (BLĬTH-fə-lee), **blithely** (BLĬTH-lee), and **blithesomely** (BLĬTH-səm-lee) *all adverbs;* **blithesomeness** (BLĬTH-səm-nis) and **blitheness** (BLĬTH-nis) *both nouns.*

bodacious (boh-DAY-shəs)

From English dialectical **bowldacious,** meaning "brazen."

1. thorough; unmistakable.

"The shepherd was known as a **bodacious** liar and champion gossip whose word could never be trusted."

2. bold; brazen.

"How could the child have turned out well when he had only the support of a **bodacious** father and a simpering mother to guide him?"

3. outstanding; remarkable.

"An hour spent waiting his turn in the barber's chair gave him enough **bodacious** yarns to fill a month's columns in the country weekly he wrote for."

Related word: **bodaciously** (boh-DAY-shəs-lee) *adverb.*

bogus (BOH-gəs)

From American, origin uncertain.

sham; spurious; counterfeit.

"Considering how much time and skill it takes to create and pass a few **bogus** ten-dollar bills, I always wonder whether he couldn't have managed his life better with a respectable job."

bombastic (bom-BAS-tik)

From English **bombast,** meaning "pretentious words," + **-ic,** an adjectival suffix meaning "in the style of."

Also given as **bombastical** (bom-BAS-ti-kəl). See also **bromidic** for further explanation of *-ic.*

of expression: high-flown, inflated, pretentious.

"Where do you suppose the brother of a monk who had taken a vow of silence gets his gift of **bombastic** oratory from?"

Related word: **bombastically** (bom-BAS-ti-kə-lee) *adverb*.

bovine (BOH-vīn)
From Latin *bovinus*, from *bos*, meaning "ox or cow."

cowlike; oxlike; dull; stolid.

"The bright college student thought cows deserved their reputations for **bovine** impassivity because they would deliver tons of milk every year without once betraying any interest in the extraction procedure."

brachycephalic. *See* **cephalic.**

bromide. *See* **bromidic.**

bromidic (broh-MID-ik)
From American **bromide**, meaning "a platitude," + **-ic**, a suffix that forms an adjective of other parts of speech; thus, for example, **poet** + **-ic** = **poetic**.

trite; platitudinous.

"Our naive hostess made the mistake of inviting the **bromidic** mayor of the town to her dinner party, only to see the other guests race through dinner in order to escape the boredom of the mayor's storytelling."

Related words: **bromide** (BROH-mīd) *noun;* **bromidically** (broh-MID-i-kə-lee) *adverb*.

bulimia. *See* **bulimic.**

bulimic (byoo-LIM-ik)
From Greek *boulimia*, meaning "great hunger."

Also given as **bulimiac** (byoo-LIM-ee-AK).

affected by uncontrollable pathological craving for food.

"Spells of food binging, followed by retching and vomiting, and then more eating were characteristic of his **bulimic** patients."

Related word: **bulimia** (byoo-LIM-ee-ə) *noun*.

bumptious (BUMP-shəs)
From English **bump** + **-tious,** an adjectival suffix.

obtrusively and noisily self-assertive.

"We may be offended by **bumptious** young people who think they are the center of the world, but we cannot help being amused by their antics."

Related words: **bumptiously** (BUMP-shəs-lee) *adverb*; **bumptiousness** (BUMP-shəs-nis) *noun*.

Bunyanesque (BUN-yə-NESK)

From the name of Paul Bunyan, a legendary lumberjack in American social history; and from the name of John Bunyan, seventeenth-century preacher and author of the allegory *Pilgrim's Progress*.

1. alluding to Paul Bunyan: of the fantastic size and unlikely exploits of characters in Paul Bunyan's legends.

"Returning combat veterans have been known to devise exaggerated accounts of their **Bunyanesque** exploits that had really been accomplished by others."

2. alluding to John Bunyan: suggestive of the allegorical writings of John Bunyan.

"To hear Edmund speak of his **Bunyanesque** climb through the Slough of Despond to the top of the literary world, we were asked to believe he had conquered almost insurmountable obstacles without any help."

C

cacophonic. *See* cacophonous.

cacophonous (kə-KOF-ə-nəs)

> From Greek *kakophónos*, from *caco-* meaning "bad" + *phone*, meaning "speech sound" + suffix *-ous*, together meaning "having bad speech sound."

> The English adjective is also given as **cacophonic** (KAK-ə-FON-ik).

> harsh; discordant.

>> "The **cacophonous** sounds ground out by our school's junior symphony and identified mysteriously as 'the music of Wagner,' constitute a general invitation to leave the auditorium."

>> Related words: **cacophonously** (kə-KOF-ə-nəs-lee) *adverb*; **cacophony** (kə-KOF-ə-nee) *noun*.

caduceus. *See* caducous.

caducous (kə-DOO-kəs)

> From Latin *caducus*, meaning "transitory or falling"; from verb *cadere*, meaning "to fall."

> Not to be confused with **caduceus** (kə-DOO-see-əs), a noun that derives from the Latin *caduceum* and Greek *karykeion*, both meaning "a herald's wand," adopted as the emblem of the medical profession.

> fleeting; transitory; perishable; falling off before the usual time.

>> "People once were said to have lived more than three score and ten years, but the emergence of certain untreatable infections has rendered our lives **caducous**."

>> Related word: **caducity** (kə-DOO-si-tee) *noun*.

calcareous (kal-KAIR-ee-əs)

From Latin *calcarius,* meaning "of lime."

chalky; containing calcium carbonate.

"British farmers raising crops on **calcareous** land sometimes find that their ancient forebears carved soil away, revealing scatological figures underneath."

Related words: **calcareously** (kal-KAIR-ee-əs-lee) *adverb;* **calcareousness** (kal-KAIR-ee-əs-nis) *noun.*

calliope. *See* **calliopean.**

calliopean (kə-LĪ-ə-PEE-ən)

From American **calliope,** meaning "steam organ," from Greek *kalliópé,* meaning "beautiful-voiced." Circus fans know this as a stretch of the imagination.

piercingly loud; imitative of a calliope.

"Only one song was known by the inventor of the machine we marched behind in those days, a screeching, **calliopean** version of *Stars and Stripes.*"

Related word: **calliope** (kə-LĪ-ə-pee) noun

callipygian (KAL-ə-PIJ-ee-ən)

From Greek *kallipygos,* meaning "having beautiful buttocks"; from *kalli-* "beautiful" + pyge "rump," + *-os* an adjectival suffix.

The adjective is also given as **callipygous** (KAL-ə-PĪ-gəs).

having shapely buttocks.

"Mr. Lorimer's criteria for engaging new secretaries were based on their **callipygian** gifts rather than their office skills."

callow (KAL-oh)

From Old English *calu,* meaning "bald." Just as early in its life an unfledged bird is bald—featherless.

inexperienced; immature.

"What more can you expect of a **callow** youth who has never had much contact with the real world?"

Related word: **callowness** (KAL-oh-nis) *noun.*

calumnious (kə-LUM-nee-əs)

From Latin *calumniosus,* meaning "full of tricks."

defamatory; slanderous; given to making malicious statements.

"Crawford habitually fabricates **calumnious** claims that cast his opponents in a bad light and win elections."

Related words: **calumniously** (kə-LUM-nee-əs-lee) *adverb*; **calumniatory** (kə-LUM-nee-ə-TOR-ee) *adjective*; **calumny** (KAL-əm-nee), **calumniation** (kə-LUM-nee-AY-shən), and **calumniator** (kə-LUM-nee-AY-tər) *all nouns*; **calumniate** (kə-LUM-nee-AYT) *verb*.

campestral (kam-PES-trəl)
From Latin *campestris*, meaning "flat"; from *campus*, meaning "field" + *-estris*, an adjectival suffix.

rural; rustic; pertaining to fields or open country.

"Sonja carried a beautiful **campestral** bouquet, all the flowers looking as though they had just been cut from living wild plants growing by the wayside as the bridal party traveled in horse-drawn coach toward the site of the wedding."

Cantabrigian (KAN-tə-BRIJ-ee-ən)
From Latin *Cantabrigia*, meaning "Cambridge."

1. of Cambridge, England; or of Cambridge University.

"I have been told that **Cantabrigian** undergraduates no longer are required to sport their traditional academic gowns."

2. of Cambridge, Massachusetts; or of Harvard University.

"Years ago, a **Cantabrigian** law-school class in Massachusetts always accepted a goodly number of City College alumni, who were sought after because of their established academic ability."

caprine (KAP-rīn)
From Latin adjective *caprinus*, from *caper*, meaning "he-goat."

goatlike; of or pertaining to goats.

"Following an introductory lecture on animal mating, we were treated to an hour-long film of **caprine** copulation that put most of us to sleep."

captious (KAP-shəs)
From Middle English *capcious*, from Latin *captiosus*, meaning "deceptive; dangerous; captious."

1. faultfinding; inclined to overstress one's faults and to make objections.

"His **captious** nature did nothing to endear him to his classmates or his teachers."

2. calculated to perplex, especially to trap an adversary in argument.

"Her **captious** questions usually bore no resemblance to the gist of a discussion under way but were meant to ensnare an opponent unversed in the intricacies of a topic."

Related words: **captiously** (KAP-shəs-lee) *adverb*; **captiousness** (KAP-shəs-nis) *noun*.

caries. *See* **cariogenic.**

cariogenic (KAR-ee-ə-JEN-ik)

From English **caries,** from Latin *caries,* meaning "decay"; + the suffix *-genic,* meaning "producing."

promoting development of tooth decay.

"By the time Jose reached adolescence, potent **cariogenic** factors had done their work, and he was told he would have to suffer many hours in a dentist's chair."

Related words: **caries** (KAIR-eez) and **cariogenicity** (KAIR-ee-oh-jə-NIS-i-tee) *both nouns*; **carious** (KAIR-ee-əs) *adjective*.

carminative (kahr-MIN-ə-tiv)

From Latin *carminatus,* past participle of infinitive *carminare,* meaning "to card (an animal's wool)."

having the quality of expelling gas from the bowel or stomach.

"Cowboys subsisting on a diet of baked beans and little else showed no amazement that they openly discussed the **carminative** quality of their boring rations."

carnivorous (kahr-NIV-ər-əs)

From Latin *carnivorus,* meaning "flesh-eating."

flesh-eating; meat-eating.

"Decreases in the number of **carnivorous** people and accompanying increases in the number of vegetarians have been mentioned by most observers."

Related words: **carnivore** (KAHR-nə-VOR), **carnivorism** (kahr-NIV-ə-rizm), and **carnivorousness** (kahr-NIV-ə-rəs-nis) *all nouns*; **carnivorously** (kahr-NIV-ə-rəs-lee) *adverb*.

caseous (KAY-see-əs)

From Latin *caseus,* meaning "cheese" + *-ous,* an adjectival suffix meaning "possessing."

of or like cheese.

"She said the cheese I had bought had an unforgivably **caseous** stench and would not allow it in the house."

casuistic (KAZH-oo-IS-tik)

From Spanish *casuista*, meaning "casuistry," from Latin *casus*, meaning "a fall."

The adjective is also given as **casuistical** (KAZH-oo-IS-ti-kəl).

overly subtle; intellectually dishonest.

"I ask you to forego your **casuistic** observations, which confuse me and your classmates."

Related words: **casuistically** (KAZH-oo-IS-ti-kə-lee) *adverb*; **casuist** (KAZH-oo-ist) and **casuistry** (KAZH-oo-ə-stree) *both nouns*.

casuistry. *See* **casuistic.**

catholic (KATH-ə-lik)

From Latin *catholicus*, from Greek *katholikós*, both meaning "universal." Sometimes capitalized. See definition 2 below.

1. wide-ranging (in interests); universal in scope.

"You will find that many of your teachers are **catholic** in their tastes and willing to read papers on any subject related to the content of their courses."

2. usually capitalized: pertaining to all Christian peoples.

"The New World soon broadened the definitions of **Catholic** to encompass Christian churches of various practices and disparate ethnic groups."

Related words: **catholicly** (kə-THOL-ik-lee) *adverb*; **catholicness** (KATH-ə-lik-nis), **catholicalness** (kə-THOL-ik-əl-nis), and **catholicity** (KATH-ə-LIS-i-tee) *all nouns*.

censorable. *See* **censurable.**

censurable (SEN-shər-ə-bəl)

From English **censure**, meaning "reprove."

deserving blame or censure.

"Our party's list of **censurable** acts and the punishment such acts merit are so clearly written that no one ever debates their validity."

Do not confuse **censurable** or any of its cognates with **censorable** (SEN-sə-rə-bəl) or its cognates. To **censor** is to play the role of censor, which enables a designated official, called **censor** (SEN-sər), to remove from public view any part or all of a publication, play, or the like.

To **censure,** by contrast, is to criticize or reprove vehemently or harshly. Whereas someone who **censors** is first given some kind of official status, any person may **censure.**

Related words: **censurableness** (SEN-shər-ə-bəl-nis), **censurability** (SEN-shər-ə-BIL-i-tee), and **censurer** (SEN-shər-ər) *all nouns*; **censurably** (SEN-shər-ə-blee) *adverb*; **censure** (SEN-shər) *noun* and *verb*.

centripetal (sen-TRIP-i-tl)

From Modern Latin *centripetus,* meaning "center-seeking."

tending toward the center.

"Politics has its own law of the **centripetal,** which is why candidates for high office often seek the center in imitation of senselessly spinning physical bodies."

Related words: **centripetally** (sen-TRIP-i-tə-lee) *adverb*; **centripetalism** (sen-TRIP-i-təl-izm) *noun*.

cephalic (sə-FAL-ik)

From Latin *cephalicus,* from Greek *kephalikós,* both meaning "pertaining to the head."

of the nature of a head; directed toward the head.

"Long before much knowledge was available concerning the workings of the brain, teachers of anthropology and psychology made a great stir about persons' differences in head shapes and fashioned a **cephalic** index as a means of categorizing the races of mankind."

It was thought that mankind exhibited three sizes and types of heads: **brachycephalic** (BRAK-ee-sə-FAL-ik) short-headed, **mesocephalic** (MEZ-oh-sə-FAL-ik) midway between short-headed and long-headed, and **dolichocephalic** (DOL-i-koh-sə-FAL-ik) long-headed.

ceriferous (si-RIF-ər-əs)

From Latin *cera,* meaning "wax" + *i* + *-ferous,* meaning "producing or secreting wax."

secreting or producing cerumen, or earwax.

"Any man told he is going deaf may well be afflicted with excessively **ceriferous** ears and have to put up with periodic cleansing of those organs."

chapfallen (CHAP-FAW-lən)

From a former English noun **chap,** meaning "lower jaw," + the adjective **fallen.**

The word is also given as **chopfallen** (CHOP-FAW-lən), characterizing dispirited or dejected persons with their lower jaws hanging loosely.

mentally depressed; dejected; chagrined.

"Once the initial results of the election were posted, the winning candidates were ebullient and most losers were **chapfallen.**"

chary (CHAIR-ee)

From Middle English and Old English *cearig,* meaning "sorrowful" and their linguistic descendants, finally reaching German *karg,* meaning "scanty."

1. wary; discreetly cautious because of apparent risks.

"Many of the **chary** children disappointed their parents by refusing outright to enter the gloomy caves the family had traveled so far to see."

2. disinclined; discreetly cautious because of inherent slowness in granting compliments, etc.

"When the old coach also proved **chary** of writing a letter of commendation, it was obvious Emily would have to look elsewhere for a sponsor."

Related words: **charily** (CHAIR-i-lee) *adverb;* **chariness** (CHAIR-ee-nis) *noun.*

cheeseparing (CHEEZ-pair-ing)

From English **cheese** + **paring,** meaning "trimming."

parsimonious; miserly.

"I soon had all I could of his **cheeseparing** ways, surely acquired from both his parents, as I found out during a miserable afternoon spent with two of the cheapest old people I had ever met."

Related word: **cheeseparer** (CHEEZ-pair-er) *noun.*

chimerical (kī-MER-i-kəl)

From English **chimera,** literally meaning "she-goat," + **-ical,** a suffix used to form adjectives from nouns.

The adjective is also given as **chimeric** (kī-MER-ik).

whimsical; given to fantastic schemes; unreal, imaginary; wildly fanciful.

"As usual, the best he could offer was a **chimerical** explanation of exactly how an ordinary goat had been induced to make its own way to the peaked roof of a twelve-story building."

Related words: **chimerically** (kī-MER-i-klee) *adverb*; **chimera** (kī-MEER-ə) *noun*.

cholera. *See* **choleric.**

choleric (KOL-ər-ik)
From Middle English *colerik*, from Latin *colericus*, from Greek *cholerikós*, all meaning "bilious."

irascible; hot-tempered; quick to fly off the handle.

"His **choleric** disposition scarcely subsided over the years until after his emergency heart bypass operation."

Related words: **cholera** (KOL-ər-ə) and **cholericness** (KOL-ər-ik-nis) *both nouns*; **cholerically** (KOL-ər-i-klee) *adverb*.

chopfallen. *See* **chapfallen.**

chthonian (THOH-nee-ən)
From Greek *chthónios*, meaning "beneath the earth."

The adjective is also given as **chthonic** (THON-ik).

dwelling in or under the surface of the earth.

"Jerry seemed convinced that in an earlier life he had been one of many **chthonian** spirits whom he would rejoin once he died."

churlish (CHUR-lish)
From Middle English and from Old English *ceorl*, meaning "man."

1. rude, vulgar, boorish; mean; ungracious; surly.

"Nobody was willing to accept **churlish** people like him who never missed a chance to act insultingly."

2. of soil: intractable; hard to work with.

"How he longed for the rich loam of the old country instead of the **churlish** hardpan he had to face every day of his arduous life in the New World."

Related words: **churlishly** (CHUR-lish-lee) *adverb*; **churl** (churl) and **churlishness** (CHUR-lish-nis) *both nouns*.

cinereous (si-NEER-ee-əs)

From Latin *cinereus,* meaning "ash-colored."

The adjective is also given as **cineritious** (SIN-ə-RISH-əs).

1. reduced to ashes; ashen.

"In less than an hour fire had reduced the shed and its contents to a **cinereous** residue."

2. ash-colored; grayish.

"No matter how hard I tried I was unable to see, much less photograph, the slender **cinereous** bird."

Related words: **cinerarium** (SIN-ə-RAIR-ee-əm) *noun;* **cinerary** (SIN-ə-RAIR-ee) *adjective.*

circumjacent (SUR-kəm-JAY-sənt)

From Latin present participle of *circumjacere,* meaning "to lie around, border on."

surrounding; lying or situated around.

"What centuries before us had been a town with vast green **circumjacent** fields was now a sooty slum residue of coal-hungry industries that had departed generations ago."

Related words: **circumjacency** (SUR-kəm-JAY-sən-see) and **circumjacence** (SUR-kəm-JAY-səns) *both nouns.*

clandestine (klan-DES-tin)

From Latin *clandestinus,* meaning "secret."

secret; private, implying deception.

"It was understood that the entire operation would be **clandestine,** since the safety of an infantry battalion lay in the balance."

Related words: **clandestinely** (klan-DES-tin-lee) *adverb;* **clandestineness** (klan-DES-tin-nis) *noun.*

claustral (KLAW-strəl)

From Latin *claustrum,* meaning "cloister," from *claustra,* meaning "bolt or lock."

cloisterlike; pertaining to a cloister.

"A kind of **claustral** solemnity pervaded the house she lived in, making for an unnatural silence among her entire family."

climactic (klī-MAK-tik)

From English **climax,** meaning "highest point," from Greek *kliméx,* meaning "ladder."

The adjective is also given as **climactical** (klī-MAK-ti-kəl).

Climactic is included here because it is often mistakenly confused with **climatic** (klī-MAT-ik), an adjective that concerns climate, not a climax. What happens is that the middle consonant "c" in **climactic** often goes unvoiced, and listeners are not certain whether **climactic** or **climatic** is intended.

Speakers of English are freely distributed between those who never make this mistake and those who regularly do.

relating to or coming to a climax.

"Engraved on my memory is the **climactic** spectacle of a lone runner in an Olympic marathon managing to finish long after darkness had fallen, facing spectators who had waited hours to be able to see a singular display of courage and heroism for love of country."

Related word: **climactically** (klī-MAK-ti-kə-lee) *adverb.*

climatic. *See* **climactic.**

clinquant (KLING-kənt)

From French *clinquant,* meaning "flashy," present participle of *clinquer,* "to clink."

spangled; tinseled; garishly ornamented.

"The matron made her appearance at the awards ceremony in an unbelievably **clinquant** gown embroidered with thousands of rhinestones and gold sequins."

cliquish (KLEE-kish)

From English **clique,** meaning "belonging to a coterie."

The adjective is also given as **cliquey** or **cliquy,** both pronounced (KLEE-kee).

as a term of reproach: accepting only members of a select group.

"Their **cliquish** exclusion extended to anyone who had not been thrown out of or at least once attended a fashionable Eastern prep school."

Related words: **cliqueless** (KLEEK-lis) *adjective;* **cliquishly** (KLEE-kish-lee) *adverb;* **clique** (kleek), **cliquism** (KLEEK-izm), and **cliquishness** (KLEE-kish-nis) *all nouns.*

cloying (KLOY-ing)

From English **cloy,** meaning "satiate," + **-ing,** a suffix forming the present participles of verbs, often used as participial adjectives.

From Middle English *acloyen,* from Latin *inclavare,* meaning "to nail in."

1. satiating; tending to cause disgust through excess.

"Above all, he seeks to wring out of his verse every last vestige of the **cloying** religiosity that usually besets him."

2. overly sentimental or ingratiating.

"In a failed attempt to show genuine interest in the young man, Felicia came through as a transparently **cloying** middle-aged mother-of-the-bride-over-your-dead-body."

Related word: **cloyingly** (KLOY-ing-lee) *adverb.*

cockamamie (KOK-ə-MAY-mee)

From American slang, an alteration of **decalcomania** (di-KAL-kə-MAY-nee-ə), meaning literally "a means of transferring pictures from specially prepared paper to another surface."

ridiculous, implausible; pointlessly complicated.

"Only a feeble-minded person standing on his head could have created the **cockamamie** organization chart my new supervisor just distributed."

cogent (KOH-jənt)

From Latin present participle *cogens* of *cogere,* an infinitive meaning "to drive together."

1. telling; powerful; convincing because of effective presentation.

"By the time she had completed her **cogent** plea for the release of the accused man, there wasn't a doubt in the world that he was innocent, nor was there a dry eye in the audience."

2. pertinent; relevant; to the point.

"Everything the woman said was **cogent** up to the time when she offered to answer any questions from the audience, questions she knew nothing about and scarcely understood."

Related words: **cogently** (KOH-jənt-lee) *adverb*; **cogency** (KOH-jən-see) *noun*.

cognoscible (kog-NOS-ə-bəl)

From Latin *cognoscere*, meaning "to know."

knowable; capable of being known.

"How many times in the history of mankind have wise men declared nothing remains in the physical world that is **cognoscible?**"

Related word: **cognoscibility** (kog-NOS-ə-BIL-i-tee) *noun*.

coltish (KOHL-tish)

From English **colt,** meaning "young horse" + adjectival suffix **-ish.**

resembling a young horse; wild, frisky, untamed; frolicsome, playful.

"The last children's nurse she hired lasted less than a month because of the twins' **coltish** behavior, which was unacceptable to their parents as well as to any other reasonably intelligent adult."

Related words: **coltishly** (KOHL-tish-lee) *adverb*; **coltishness** (KOHL-tish-nis) *noun*.

colubrine (KOL-ə-BRĪN)

From Latin *coluber,* meaning "snakelike."

snakelike; cunning; wily; resembling a snake.

"The **colubrine** candidate had astounded us all by insinuating his way to the top in a single year without attracting undue notice."

Related word: **colubrid** (KOL-ə-brid) *noun*.

comate. *See* **comose.**

comatose (KOM-ə-TOHS)

From Greek *kôma,* meaning "sleep."

1. torpid; lacking alertness.

"My **comatose** sons understand fully the need for greater care in managing the ranch they one day will inherit."

2. affected with coma.

"After many hours in a **comatose** state, the patient appeared incapable of being roused."

Related words: **comatosely** (KOM-ə-TOHS-lee) *adverb*; **comatoseness** (KOM-ə-TOHS-nis) and **comatosity** (KOM-ə-TOS-i-tee) *both nouns*.

comestible (kə-MES-tə-bəl)

From Latin *comestibilis,* from *comedere,* meaning "to devour."

edible; eatable; fit to eat.

"Anything remotely **comestible** disappears within minutes after my voracious sons get home from school."

Related word: **comestibles** (kə-MES-tə-bəlz) *noun.*

comose (KOH-mohs)

From Latin *comosus,* meaning "shaggy"; from Greek *kóme,* meaning "hair."

The adjective is also given as **comate** (KOH-mayt).

hairy; comate, tufted.

"Gone are the days when **comose** young men brought shame upon a family when they managed to avoid sneaking into a barbershop for their semiannual shearing."

compendious (kəm-PEN-dee-əs)

From Middle English, from Latin *compendiosus,* meaning "advantageous, abridged."

succinct, concise; containing the substance of a subject in compact form.

"What they were looking for was a **compendious** treatment of all the world's best literature without having to read the originals."

Related words: **compendiously** (kəm-PEN-dee-əs-lee) *adverb;* **compendiousness** (kəm-PEN-dee-əs-nis) and **compendium** (kəm-PEN-dee-əm) *both nouns.*

compendium. *See* **compendious.**

complacent (kəm-PLAY-sənt)

From present participle of Latin infinitive *complacere,* meaning "to please." See the meaning of **complaisant** in the next entry.

1. self-satisfied; smug; feeling pleasure in one's own condition.

"Above all, I was warned, never show that you are **complacent** about your dog's chances of being named best in show."

2. pleasant; complaisant.

"I was entirely **complacent** about my failure to win a medal in the competition until I saw that the two leaders were faced with suspension for interference with one another during the race."

Related words: **complacently** (kəm-PLAY-sənt-lee) *adverb*; **complacency** (kəm-PLAY-sən-see) and **complacence** (kəm-PLAY-səns) *both nouns.*

complaisant (kəm-PLAY-sənt)

From French *complaisance*, present participle of *complaire*; from present participle of Latin *complacere*, both the French and Latin infinitives meaning "to please."

There is less feeling of smugness in **complaisant** than there is in **complacent,** even though the meanings of the two words are coming together.

agreeable, obliging, accommodating; disposed to please; hypocritically indifferent to strict moral standards.

"The child's **complaisant** ways did not go unnoticed, I am glad to say, even though good manners in the young are often overlooked."

Related words: **complaisantly** (kəm-PLAY-sənt-lee) *adverb*; **complaisance** (kəm-PLAY-səns) *noun.*

compunction. *See* **compunctious.**

compunctious (kəm-PUNGK-shəs)

From English **compunction,** meaning "contrition or remorse."

regretful; remorseful; causing or feeling compunction.

"Although Jane had no part in the botched plot, I cannot see why she insists on feeling **compunctious** about it."

Related words: **compunctiously** (kəm-PUNGK-shəs-lee) *adverb*; **compunctionless** (kəm-PUNGK-shən-lis) *adjective*; **compunction** (kəm-PUNGK-shən) *noun.*

concinnous (kən-SIN-əs)

From Latin *concinnus*, meaning "symmetrical, polished."

agreeable, harmonious; elegant, graceful.

"Ethel was well liked and admired by her coworkers for her **concinnous** manners."

Related words: **concinnity** (kən-SIN-i-tee) *noun*; **concinnate** (KON-sə-NAYT) *verb.*

concupiscent (kon-KYOO-pi-sənt)

From Latin *concupiscens*, present participle of *concupiscere*, meaning "to covet, desire, long for (someone)."

lustful; eagerly desirous.

"Plato, the lecturer said, saw the soul at the same time as rational, impatient, and **concupiscent,** giving us a further indication of the complexity of human emotions as seen in ancient Greece."

Related words: **concupiscence** (kon-KYOO-pi-səns) *noun*; **concupiscible** (kon-KYOO-pi-sə-bəl) *adjective.*

condign (kən-DĪN)

From Latin *condignus,* meaning "very worthy."

well deserved; appropriate; fitting.

"Because of the severity of the crimes committed, the prisoner's sentence satisfied us as being **condign.**"

Related words: **condignly** (kən-DĪN-lee) *adverb*; **condignity** (kən-DIG-ni-tee) and **condignness** (kən-DĪN-nis) *both nouns.*

congruent. *See* **congruous.**

congruous (KONG-groo-əs)

From Latin *congruus,* meaning "agreeable."

The adjective is also given as **congruent** (KONG-groo-ənt).

suitable; conformable; appropriate, coherent; meeting requirements; being in agreement or harmony.

"The present international commission seems to be incapable of bringing all three nations together in a **congruous** settlement."

Related words: **congruously** (KONG-groo-əs-lee) and **congruently** (KONG-groo-ənt-lee) *both adverbs*; **congruousness** (KONG-groo-əs-nis), **congruity** (kən-GROO-i-tee), **congruence** (KONG-groo-əns), and **congruency** (KONG-groo-ən-see) *all nouns.*

consanguineous (KON-sang-GWIN-ee-əs)

From Latin *consanguineus,* meaning "of the same blood." (In Latin, the noun *blood* is given as *sanguis.*)

The adjective is also given as **consanguine** (kon-SANG-gwin) and **consanguineal** (kon-sang-GWIN-ee-əl).

of the same blood; having the same ancestry.

"Almost every society, from the least advanced to the most highly sophisticated, has a taboo on **consanguineous** marriage, which prevents siblings and cousins from intermarrying."

Related words: **consanguineously** (KON-sang-GWIN-ee-əs-lee) *adverb*; **consanguinity** (KON-sang-GWIN-i-tee) *noun*.

consuetudinary (KON-swi-TOOD-in-ER-ee)

From Latin *consuetudinarius*, adjectival form of *consuetudo*, meaning "custom, habit."

customary; traditional.

"Even in complex societies, matters of everyday life are often subject to regulation by **consuetudinary** law."

Related word: **consuetude** (KON-swi-TOOD) *noun*.

contemporaneous (kən-TEM-pə-RAY-nee-əs)

From Latin *contemporaneus*, meaning "contemporary." (In Latin, "time" is given as *tempus*.)

Contemporaneous is similar in form to **contemporary**. The essential difference between these two rests in that **contemporaneous** applies to events, and **contemporary** applies to people and the things they have, as shown below.

Contemporaneous. "Failing memory being what it is, **contemporaneous** accounts of great events usually deserve more credence than historical accounts."

Contemporary. "Franklin D. Roosevelt is remembered affectionately by most **contemporary** journalists, politicians, and statesmen."

said of events: existing or occurring during the same time; belonging to the same period.

"Long experience with the unreliability of recalled testimony forced the attorney to seek witnesses who could give good **contemporary** accounts of the crime."

Related words: **contemporaneously** (kən-TEM-pə-RAY-nee-əs-lee) *adverb*; **contemporaneity** (kən-TEM-pə-rə-NEE-i-tee) and **contemporaneousness** (kən-TEM-pə-RAY-nee-əs-nis) *both nouns*.

contemporary (kən-TEM-pə-RER-ee)

For word origin and discussion of differences in meaning, see **contemporaneous**.

1. belonging to the same time or period; living together in time.

"After much study he is still surprised to find a lack of interest among **contemporary** foreign-language newspapers in the onset of a major economic depression."

2. simultaneous; characteristic of the same time or period.

"My brother and Jonas Salk, considered representative **contemporary** physicians of their time, were completely unaware of antibiotics until after they had completed their formal studies."

3. modern; characteristic of the same period.

"The editor of our newspaper shows no interest in **contemporary** architecture, apparently considering it only an aberration."

Related words: **contemporarily** (kən-TEM-pə-RER-i-lee) *adverb*; **contemporariness** (kən-TEM-pə-RER-i-nes); **contemporize** (kən-TEM-pə-RĪz) *verb*.

continual (kən-TIN-yoo-əl)

From Latin *continuus*, meaning "uninterrupted," from *continere*, meaning "to hang together." Similar in form to **continuous.**

Continual and **continuous** are almost always used interchangeably, even by the best writers, yet language devotees insist on differentiating the troublesome pair.

The definitions given in the remainder of this entry, **continual,** and the next entry, **continuous,** begin by showing the strict interpretation of young writers and academics and end with a relaxed attitude.

Continual. Characterized by occasional pauses, as though to regroup: "After not being heard for a few hours, there he was again, with his **continual** yawping."

1. frequently recurring; often repeating, intermittent.

"My daughter's **continual** tears got her nowhere and were soon replaced by dry-eyed smiles."

2. unceasing; incessant; always; perpetual.

"**Continual** presence of one or more adults is now a requirement in day schools."

Related words: **continually** (kən-TIN-yoo-ə-lee) *adverb*; **continuable** (kən-TIN-yoo-ə-bəl) *adjective*; **continuality** (kən-TIN-yoo-AL-i-tee), **continuance** (kən-TIN-yoo-əns), **continuation** (kən-TIN-yoo-AY-shən), and **continualness** (kən-TIN-yoo-əl-nis) *all nouns*; **continue** (kən-TIN-yoo) *verb*.

continuous (kə-TIN-yoo-əs)

From Latin *continuus*, meaning "uninterrupted," from *continere*, meaning "to hang together."

The English adjective is also given as **continued** (kən-TIN-yood) and **continual.**

Continuous. Never pausing, not even for a moment: "How happy I was to hear once again the **continuous** roar of Niagara Falls, knowing the torrent would not slow to a trickle in the lifetime of my granddaughter."

1. ceaseless; uninterrupted in time.

"We had to put up with **continuous** dialing and ringing every day when the children were home from school."

2. unbroken; never ending.

"I am seeking a high-fidelity machine that will play a **continuous** tape."

Related words: **continuously** (kən-TIN-yoo-əs-lee) *adverb*; **continuousness** (kən-TIN-yoo-əs-nis) and **continuum** (kən-TIN-yoo-əm) *both nouns.*

contumacious (KON-tuu-MAY-shəs)
From Latin *contumax*, meaning "obstinate."

stubbornly perverse; insubordinate, rebellious.

"His **contumacious** behavior is disrupting the smooth operation of the company."

Related words: **contumaciously** (KON-too-MAY-shəs-lee) *adverb*; **contumacy** (KON-too-mə-see), **contumaciousness** (KON-too-MAY-shəs-nis), and **contumacity** (KON-too-MAS-i-tee) *all nouns.*

contumelious (KON-too-MEE-lee-əs)
From Latin noun *contumelia*, meaning "invective; an insult, a libel."

displaying contempt in words or actions; tending to convey humiliation.

"They expressed themselves in such **contumelious** language during the negotiation that we wondered if they were trying to sabotage us."

Related words: **contumely** (KON-tuu-mə-lee) and **contumeliousness** (KON-too-MEE-lee-əs-nis) *both nouns*; **contumeliously** (KON-too-MEE-lee-əs-lee) *adverb.*

coriaceous (KOR-ee-AY-shəs)
From Late Latin *coriaceus*, meaning "leathern": from Latin *corium*, meaning "hide, leather."

resembling leather.

"Years of exposure to the sun left him with weather-beaten, **coriaceous** skin that identified him as a true cowboy and made him a favorite with all the impressionable young women guests."

corrigible (KOR-i-jə-bəl)
From Latin *corrigere*, meaning "to correct."

The English word **corrigible** is much better known in its antonym **incorrigible,** which doesn't say much for our social structure.

1. rectifiable; capable of being corrected.

"Many heretofore lethal medical conditions are now **corrigible** by surgical intervention or by antibiotics."

2. of faults: capable of being amended, improved, or reformed.

"The new warden brought to his job the hope and possibility that all crimes were **corrigible.**"

3. of persons: open to correction.

"The child's parents long ago decided he was not **corrigible** and sent him off to a so-called military prep school."

Related words: **corrigibly** (KOR-ri-jə-blee) *adverb;* **corrigibility** (KOR-ri-jə-BIL-i-tee) and **corrigibleness** (KOR-ri-jə-bəl-nis) *both nouns.*

coruscant (kə-RUS-kənt)
From Latin infinitive *coruscare*, meaning "to flash, quiver."

scintillating; coruscating; sparkling or gleaming.

"The star's splendid, **coruscant** gown reflected the brilliant lights of Oscar night and brought rounds of applause as she made her way into the theater."

Related words: **coruscate** (KOR-ə-skayt) *verb;* **coruscation** (KOR-ə-SKAY-shən) *noun.*

corvine (KOR-vīn)
From Latin *corvinus*, meaning "a crow."

resembling or pertaining to a crow.

"Ornithologists have observed that **corvine** birds are susceptible to heretofore unobserved fatal viral infections."

corybantic (KOR-ə-BAN-tik)
From Latin and Greek *Corybas*, a mythologic spirit given to wildness.

Also given as **Corybantian** (KOR-ə-BAN-shən) and **Corybantine** (KOR-ə-BAN-tin).

unrestrained; frenzied.

"Late in the evening of heavy imbibing, the band broke into a wild number and the crowd worked itself up into a traditional **corybantic** dance the local people had not seen the match of in years."

costive (KOS-tiv)

From Middle English *costif* through intermediate European languages back to Latin *constipatus*, meaning "tightfisted" as well as "constipated."

Constipatus is a past participle of *constipare*, literally meaning "to crowd or press together." A beautiful example of linguistic imagination.

1. constipated; suffering from hardness and retention of feces.

"The patient complained he was occasionally **costive,** but when told he should have a colonoscopy, he refused, saying all he wanted was a prescription for an effective laxative."

2. reticent; slow or reluctant to act or to express opinions.

"Our team could never decide whether Sean was slow-witted or merely **costive,** but they did know they needed a coach who was more assertive."

Related words: **costively** (KOS-tiv-lee) *adverb*; **costiveness** (KOS-tiv-nis) *noun*.

couth (kooth)

A back formation from the more popular English word **uncouth,** meaning "unsophisticated; lacking in polish."

sophisticated; refined; polished.

"No one seems to know where a hayseed like him could have learned his manners—he was even known to kiss ladies' hands—but there was no doubt his **couth** behavior was in sharp contrast to that of country bumpkins."

crapulent. *See* **crapulous.**

crapulous (KRAP-yə-ləs)

From Latin *crapula*, meaning "drunkenness"; from Greek *kraipále*, meaning "drunkenness, hangover."

Also given as **crapulent** (KRAP-yə-lənt).

While some lexicographers try hard to differentiate the meanings of the adjectives **crapulent** and **crapulous,** nothing is gained by this pursuit. Drunk is drunk. And hung over is hung over.

1. intemperate; inclined to drunkenness or overeating.

"Monthly dinners with his **crapulous** friends invariably led to excessive consumption of rich food and strong drink."

2. suffering ill effects of such excess; resulting from drunkenness.

"The **crapulous** hangovers, pounding headaches, and wrenching nausea made him certain it was time he became a teetotaler."

Related words: **crapulously** (KRAP-yə-ləs-lee) *adverb;* **crapulence** (KRAP-yə-ləns), **crapulency** (KRAP-yə-lən-see), and **crapulousness** (KRAP-you-ləs-nis) *all nouns.*

credible. *See* **credulous.**

credulous (KREJ-ə-ləs)

From Latin *credulus,* meaning "trusting," from *credere,* meaning "to believe."

Not to be confused with **credible** (KRED-ə-bəl), meaning "believable, trustworthy"; incompetent newscasters commonly make this mistake.

1. of a person: gullible; disposed to believe too readily.

"I was exasperated by my **credulous** mother's ready acceptance of everything she read in the daily newspaper."

2. of things: arising from trusting too readily.

"The police procedure was sufficiently **credulous** that the detectives were willing to let him go free even though several witnesses claimed they had seen him commit the crime."

Related words: **credulously** (KREJ-ə-ləs-lee) *adverb;* **credulousness** (KREJ-ə-ləs-nis) and **credulity** (krə-DOO-li-tee) *both nouns.*

crepuscular (kri-PUS-kyə-lər)

From English **crepuscule,** meaning "twilight, dusk"; from Latin *crepusculum,* of the same meanings, from the Latin adjective *creper,* meaning "dark, doubtful."

dim; of or resembling twilight.

"As I sat at my desk and wrote, I could only summon up unsatisfactory **crepuscular** images of my formative years."

Related words: **crepuscule** (kri-PUS-kyool) and **crepuscle** (kri-PUS-əl) *both nouns.*

cunctative (KUNGK-tə-tiv)

From Latin *cunctatio,* meaning "delay"; from *cunctatus,* meaning "hesitated," past participle of *cunctari* "to delay."

dilatory; procrastinative; prone to delay.

"After three years of his brand of leadership, we have become so accustomed to his **cunctative** style that notions of efficiency have all but vanished from our discourse."

Related words: **cunctatious** (kungk-TAY-shəs) and **cunctatory** (KUNGK-tə-TOR-ee) *both adjectives;* **cunctator** (kungk-TAY-tər) and **cunctatorship** (kungk-TAY-tər-SHIP) *both nouns.*

cuneal (KYOO-nee-əl)

From Latin *cuneatus,* meaning "wedge-shaped"; from *cuneus,* meaning "wedge."

The adjective is also given as **cuneate** (KYOO-nee-it).

cuneiform; wedge-shaped.

"Her mysteriously marked **cuneal** cookies, labeled 'Egyptian Mummy Cookies,' put off some superstitious customers."

Related words: **cuneated** (KYOO-nee-AYT-id), **cuneatic** (KYOO-nee-AT-ik), and **cuneiform** (kyoo-NEE-ə-FORM) *all adjectives.*

cupreous (KYOO-pree-əs)

From Latin *cupreus,* meaning "of copper."

copperlike; resembling copper; copper-colored; reddish-brown; containing or consisting of copper.

"Our place is high above a stream cutting through a valley that is said to be **cupreous,** but no one has tried to mine there in many years."

Related words: **cupric** (KYOO-prik), **cuprous** (KYOO-prəs), and **cupriferous** (kyoo-PRIF-ər-əs) *all adjectives.*

curmudgeonly (kər-MUJ-ən-lee)

Derivation unknown beyond the English noun **curmudgeon,** meaning "a miser or stingy person."

Those meanings and the adjectival meanings, known by the editors of the *Oxford English Dictionary* to have existed from the sixteenth century into the nineteenth, led to the following.

difficult; cantankerous; bad-tempered.

"Some persons forgive his **curmudgeonly** behavior by saying he had an unhappy childhood or is in a bad marriage, but I think he was just born mean."

cyaneous (sī-AN-ee-əs)

From Latin *cyaneus,* from Greek *kyáneos,* from *kyános,* meaning "dark blue."

of the color deep blue; azure.

"The pretty young girl's **cyaneous** eyes reminded me of the sky on a clear day."

Related word: **cyanic** (sī-AN-ik) *adjective.*

D

daedal (DEED-l)

From Latin *daedalus,* from Greek *daídalos,* both meaning "skillful."

Also from Daedalus, of Greek mythology. This skilled artificer constructed the Cretan labyrinth and made wings for himself and his son Icarus to enable them to escape from Crete.

1. skillful; ingenious.

"Try as I would, the conjurer's **daedal** finger work with cards had me thoroughly confused in no time at all."

2. marvelously intricate.

"I managed to spend half an hour examining Sophie's prize-winning comforter, which displayed her **daedal** stitchery."

Related words: **Daedalian** and **Daedalean** (both di-DAY-lee-ən), and **Daedalic** (di-DAL-ik) *all adjectives.*

dastardly (DAS-tərd-lee)

From English **dastard,** about which little more is known.

The adjective is also given as **dastard** (DAS-tərd).

1. of a person: cowardly; sneaking.

"About the only thing you can be sure of is that a **dastardly** companion will never change the baseness of his ways."

2. of an act: pusillanimous; showing cowardice.

"Desertion at the first sign of danger showed clearly the **dastardly** behavior we could expect of the likes of him."

Related words: **dastard** (DAS-tərd) and **dastardliness** (DAS-tərd-lee-nis) *both nouns;* **dastardly** (DAS-tərd-lee) *also adverb.*

daunting (DAWN-ting)

See Latin origin given below for **dauntless.**

frightful; intimidating; disheartening; discouraging.

"Most important of all the things they were told prior to the invasion was to be ready to stand together and fight off anything enemy propagandists would say about the **daunting** battle they were about to face."

Related words: **dauntingly** (DAWN-ting-lee) *adverb*; **dauntingness** (DAWN-ting-nis) *noun*.

dauntless (DAWNT-lis)

From English **daunt,** meaning "to intimidate"; from Latin *domitare,* meaning "to conquer."

While you and I aspire to be **dauntless** rather than have to face a **daunting** world, we both know that the two words come from the same Latin source.

intrepid; indomitable; fearless; not to be intimidated.

"By his actions during the initial assault on the enemy-held hill, our **dauntless** leader somehow was able to stir his troops to valor previously unsurpassed in the history of the division."

Related words: **daunt** (dawnt) *verb*; **dauntlessly** (DAWNT-lis-lee) *adverb*; **dauntlessness** (DAWNT-lis-nis) *noun*.

decalcomania. *See* **cockamamie.**

decamerous (di-KAM-ər-əs)

From Latin *deca,* meaning "ten," + -*merous,* a combining form meaning "having parts": together, "ten-parted."

having ten divisions or parts.

"The dreary **decamerous** story was ideally suited for inducing sleep in overcharged young campers."

Related words, in homage to Boccaccio: **Decameron** (di-KAM-ər-ən) *noun*; **Decameronic** (di-KAM-ə-RON-ik) *adjective*.

declivitous (di-KLIV-i-təs)

From Latin *declivitas,* meaning "sloping ground."

having a somewhat steep or considerably downward slope.

"I will never again buy a house that is cursed with a **declivitous** driveway, no matter how attractive the price."

Related words: **declivity** (di-KLIV-i-tee) *noun*; **declivous** (di-KLĪV-əs) and **declivent** (di-KLĪV-ənt) *both adjectives.*

decumbent (di-KUM-bənt)

From Latin *decumbens*, present participle of *decumbere*, meaning "to recline."

recumbent; lying down.

"I am told that in those days a patient hospitalized after repair of a detached retina was told to remain **decumbent** for at least two weeks before trying to get out of bed."

Related words: **decumbently** (di-KUM-bənt-lee) *adverb*; **decumbence** (di-KUM-bəns) and **decumbency** (di-KUM-bən-see) *both nouns.*

defeasible (di-FEE-zə-bəl)

From Anglo-French *defesible*, meaning "capable of being undone."

Defeasible, of course, is an antonym of the English word *feasible*, as is **indefeasible** (IN-di-FEE-zə-bəl).

capable of being terminated or annulled.

"The judge explained to the woman asking for a divorce that, once granted, the writ would not be **defeasible**."

Related words: **defease** (di-FEEZ) *verb*; **defeasance** (di-FEE-zəns), **defeasibility** (di-FEE-zi-BIL-i-tee), and **defeasibleness** (di-FEE-zi-bəl-nis) *all nouns.*

deferential (DEF-ə-REN-shəl)

From French *déférence*, meaning "showing respect."

respectful; showing deference; characterized by deference.

"Young interns were always **deferential** when dealing with their superiors."

Related words: **deferentially** (DEF-ə-REN-shə-lee) *adverb*; **deferent** (DEF-ər-ənt) *adjective*; **deference** (DEF-ər-əns) *noun.*

dégagé (day-gah-ZHAY)

From French past participle *dégagé* of infinitive *dégager*, meaning "to put at ease."

in manner: detached, unconstrained; without emotional involvement.

"While you may be inclined to be emotionally involved in the family crisis, **dégagé** behavior would be more useful."

dehiscent (di-HIS-ənt)

From Latin *dehiscere*, meaning "to gape, yawn; burst open."

in surgery: open; gaping.

"After my operation had begun to heal I was told to my dismay that my wound was **dehiscent** and had to be sewn together once more."

Related word: **dehisce** (di-HIS) *verb.*

deiform (DEE-ə-FORM)

From Latin *deus*, meaning "god," + *-formis*, a suffix meaning "having the form of."

godlike; divine; having the form or nature of a god.

"According to the minister, at that very moment the entire congregation stood as one person and vividly saw a **deiform** creature rise from the pulpit and vanish into air."

Related word: **deiformity** (DEE-ə-FORM-i-tee) *noun.*

deleterious (DEL-i-TEER-ee-əs)

From Greek *deletérios*, meaning "destructive."

1. noxious; damaging to health.

"Something she served at dinner turned out to be **deleterious,** and eventually the entire party ended up in the emergency room."

2. injurious; mentally or morally harmful.

"Tommy's parents withdrew him from the school when they decided his studies were having a **deleterious** effect on him."

Related words: **deleteriously** (DEL-i-TEER-ee-əs-lee) *adverb*; **deleteriousness** (DEL-i-TEER-ee-əs-nis) *noun*; **delete** (di-LEET) *verb*; **deletable** (di-LEET-ə-bəl) *adjective.*

Delphic (DEL-fik)

From Latin *Delphicus*, from Greek *Delphikós*, both referring to the ancient Greek city of Delphi, which was the site of an oracle of Apollo.

Delphic, also given as **Delphian** (DEL-fee-ən), means "referring to the city, to Apollo, or to the other oracles." Of greater importance for the modern reader, however, is the meaning given below.

also given as **delphic**: oracular, obscure, ambiguous.

"There is complete agreement that any **delphic** answer I give will sound intelligent but not be clearly understood."

Related word: **delphically** (DEL-fi-klee) *adverb.*

demimondaine (DEM-ee-mon-DAYN)
From French *demimonde,* literally "half-world," + *-aine,* a French adjectival suffix.

A **demimondaine,** as a noun, is a woman of the **demimonde** (DEM-ee-MOND), which is this "half-world."

concerning the half-world peopled by a class of women of doubtful reputations.

"Without being particularly aware of sliding downward in reputation, Nana found her life as a sought-after member of **demimondaine** Paris quite exciting—at least for a time."

démodé (day-maw-DAY)
From French *démodé,* past participle of *démoder,* meaning "to put out of fashion."

Also given as the more anglicized **demoded** (dee-MOH-did), with the same meaning.

out of fashion.

"Sylvia's flowered **démodé** dresses embarrassed her fashion-conscious daughters."

demotic (di-MOT-ik)
From Greek *demotikós,* meaning "popular."

1. in linguistics: vernacular; pertaining to everyday language.

"His baseball stories captured colorful American **demotic** speech in a way no other writing since has managed to do."

2. popular; pertaining to ordinary people.

"In searching for a winning presidential candidate, major parties are aware of the importance of the **demotic** personality, a trait that says to us this candidate is quite smart, but no better than you or I."

demulcent (di-MUL-sənt)
From Latin *demulcens,* present participle of *demulcere,* meaning "to stroke," from infinitive *mulcere,* meaning "to soothe."

in medicine: soothing; allaying irritation.

"About all we could do for the injured man was employ **demulcent** ointments in hope they would allay his severe irritation."

dendrophagous (den-DROF-ə-gəs)

From Latin *dendro-*, meaning "tree," + combining form *-phagous*, meaning "feeding on."

of insects: feeding on the wood of trees.

"Not until we saw clear evidence of their depredations did we know that **dendrophagous** beetles had been at work, and by then it was too late to save the trees."

dentulous (DEN-chə-ləs)

A back formation of English **edentulous,** meaning "toothless, possessing no teeth."

The key to the word is the prefix **e-,** meaning "without." Removing this prefix miraculously restores the missing teeth.

bearing or possessing teeth.

"The puppy left an ample supply of chewed shoes as evidence that he was **dentulous.**"

Related words: **dentist** (DEN-tist), **dentistry** (DEN-tə-stree), **dentition** (den-TISH-ən), **denture** (DEN-chər), and **denturism** (DEN-chə-RIZ-əm) *all nouns;* **dentoid** (DEN-toyd) *adjective.*

deprecative (DEP-ri-KAY-tiv)

From French *déprécatif* from Latin *deprecativus,* both meaning "disparaging, expressive of earnest disapproval."

Also intended by **deprecatory** (DEP-ri-kə-TOR-ee).

Both **deprecative** and **deprecatory** are related to the verb **deprecate** (DEP-ri-KAYT), which expresses the disapproving action or feelings conveyed by the two adjectives: "My opponent, obviously finding fault with everything I say or think, unsurprisingly **deprecates** every suggestion I make."

Do not confuse the verbs **depreciate** (di-PREE-shee-AYT) and **deprecate. Depreciate** means (1) make or become lower in value, as well as (2) disparage.

disparaging: serving to express disapproval.

"He was warned that **deprecative** remarks would discourage his son, whereas words of encouragement would assure the boy of support."

Related words: **deprecatively** (DEP-ri-KAY-tiv-lee), **deprecatorily** (DEP-ri-kə-TOR-i-lee), and **deprecatingly** (DEP-ri-KAYT-ing-lee) *all adverbs*; **deprecation** (DEP-ri-KAY-shən) and **deprecator** (DEP-ri-kay-tor) *both nouns*.

deprecatory *See* **deprecative.**

depreciative *See* **deprecative.**

derisive (di-RĪ-siv)

From the English noun **derision,** meaning "mockery," from Latin infinitive *deridere,* meaning "to laugh at."

The English adjective **derisive** is also given as **derisory** (di-RĪ-sə-ree), usually meaning "worthy of ridicule," as in "selling damaged books at **derisory** prices."

scoffing; contemptuous; mocking; expressing derision.

"I have been told that the cheerleaders advocate leading **derisive** cheers against the other team, thinking sophisticated spectators will perceive the cheers as mockery."

Related words: **derisively** (di-RĪ-siv-lee) *adverb*; **derisible** (di-RIZ-ə-bəl) *adjective*; **derisiveness** (di-RĪ-siv-nis) and **derision** (di-RIZH-ən) *both nouns*.

derogatory (di-ROG-ə-TOR-ee)

From Late Latin *derogatorius,* meaning "cursing."

Also given far less frequently as **derogative** (di-ROG-ə-tiv).

disparaging; disrespectful; lowering the reputation of someone.

"All the **derogatory** opinions directed toward him seemed to have no effect on his determination to pursue the coveted nomination."

Related words: **derogatorily** (di-ROG-ə-TOR-i-lee) and **derogatively** (di-ROG-ə-tiv-lee) *both adverbs*; **derogatoriness** (di-ROG-ə-TOR-ee-nis) *noun*.

desiderative (di-SID-ər-ə-tiv)

From Latin *desideratus,* past participle of *desiderare,* meaning "to require."

having or expressing desire.

"In the life he leads, he considers expensive clothing, summer cottages, and the latest restaurants **desiderative** indulgences."

Related words: **desiderate** (di-SID-ə-RAYT) *verb*; **desideratum** (di-SID-ə-RAH-təm) and **desiderium** (DES-i-DEER-ee-əm) *both nouns.*

detersive (di-TUR-siv)

From Middle French *détersif,* from Latin *detersus,* past participle of *detergere,* meaning "to clean."

Detersive is also used as a noun, meaning "a detergent."

tending to cleanse; having the quality of cleansing.

"To my surprise the **detersive** agent lived up to the wild claims made for its cleansing ability."

Related words: **detersively** (di-TUR-siv-lee) *adverb*; **detersiveness** (di-TUR-siv-nis) *noun.*

detumescent (DEE-too-MES-ənt)

From Latin infinitive *detumescere,* meaning "to become less swollen."

Antonym of **tumescent** (too-MES-ənt).

becoming less swollen, less nearly erect.

"A stand-up comic suggested that if the drug called Viagra could be such a success, there ought to be a marketing niche for a **detumescent** drug called Falls."

Related word: **detumescence** (DEE-too-MES-əns) *noun.*

dewy-eyed (DOO-ee-ID)

From English **dewy,** meaning "moist," + **eyed,** meaning "having eyes."

credulously innocent; trusting; romantically naive.

"How could you have been so cruel as to have taken advantage of a **dewy-eyed** ingenue?"

dexterous (DEK-strəs)

From Latin *dexter,* meaning "right hand." Also given as **dextrous.**

1. right-handed; adroit in the use of hands and body.

"Elaine was the most **dexterous** of the potters she knew, rarely having to discard any of her work."

2. clever; mentally acute.

"It took many years of hard work and many mistakes to become so **dexterous** in the management of her money."

Related words: **dextral** (DEK-strəl) *adjective;* **dexterously** (DEK-stər-əs-lee) *adverb;* **dexterity** (dek-STER-i-tee), **dexterousness** (DEK-strəs-nis), and **dextrality** (dek-STRAL-i-tee) *all nouns.*

diaphaneity *See* **diaphanous.**

diaphanous (dī-AF-ə-nəs)

From Medieval Latin *diaphanus,* from Greek *diaphaínen,* meaning "to show through."

pellucid, translucent; permitting passage of light and vision.

"Whether dancers intent on attracting spirited young men choose to wear **diaphanous** gowns is entirely their own decision."

Related words: **diaphanously** (dī-AF-ə-nəs-lee) *adverb;* **diaphanousness** (dī-AF-ə-nəs-nis) and **diaphaneity** (dī-AF-ə-NEE-i-tee) *both nouns.*

dichotomous (dī-KOT-ə-məs)

From Medieval Latin *dichotomos,* from Greek *dichótomos,* both meaning "cut in half."

divided or dividing into two.

"The acrimonious primary elections exposed the growing feeling that sooner or later there would be a **dichotomous** movement within each party."

Related words: **dichotomously** (dī-KOT-ə-məs-lee) *adverb;* **dichotomy** (dī-KOT-ə-mee), **dichotomousness** (dī-KOT-ə-məs-nis), **dichotomist** (dī-KOT-ə-mist), and **dichotomization** (dī-KOT-ə-mi-ZAY-shən) *all nouns;* **dichotomize** (dī-KOT-ə-MĪZ) *verb;* **dichotomistic** (dī-KOT-ə-MIS-tik) *adjective.*

diffident (DIF-i-dənt)

From Latin *diffidens,* present participle of infinitive *diffidere,* meaning "to distrust."

1. shy; timid; wanting in self-confidence.

"By accident I discovered that his **diffident** demeanor vanished when he was with friends and not with his parents."

2. restrained in manner.

"I have never been able to understand why he kept his **diffident** manner even after he had become a big Broadway star."

Related words: **diffidently** (DIF-i-dənt-lee) *adverb;* **diffidentness** (DIF-i-dənt-nis) and **diffidence** (DIF-i-dəns) *both nouns.*

dilettante (DIL-i-TAHNT)

From Italian *dilettante,* meaning "a lover of the arts"; from Latin *delectare,* meaning "to delight, amuse."

of or pertaining to those who take up an art merely as a pastime.

"Our conductor condemned absence or lateness for a rehearsal as a sign of **dilettante** indulgence that would never be acceptable among professionals."

Related words: **dilettantish** (DIL-i-TAHN-tish) *adjective;* **dilettantism** (DIL-i-tahn-TIZ-əm) *noun.*

dipsomaniacal (DIP-sə-mə-NĪ-ə-kəl)

From English **dipsomania,** meaning "alcoholism, an irresistible craving for drink"; from Greek *dipsa,* meaning "thirst," + the well-understood word **maniac.**

This term, once popular, is hardly ever heard today.

affected with alcoholism.

"Strangely enough, no one in Jerry's family drank beer, wine, or whiskey at all, yet he was **dipsomaniacal** before he left college, and died of overdrinking by the time he was thirty."

Related words: **dipsomania** (DIP-sə-MAY-nee-ə) and **dipsomaniac** (DIP-sə-MAY-nee-AK) *both nouns.*

disaffected (DIS-ə-FEK-tid)

From English **disaffect,** meaning "to estrange." A verb in the past tense and an adjective.

unfriendly, hostile, as toward government or authority.

"His former supporters became **disaffected** by his bad judgment, questionable appointments, and hints of scandal in his first administration."

Related words: **disaffectedly** (DIS-ə-FEK-tid-lee) *adverb;* **disaffectedness** (DIS-ə-FEK-tid-nis) and **disaffection** (DIS-ə-FEK-shən) *both nouns;* **disaffect** (DIS-ə-FEKT) *verb.*

discommodious (DIS-kə-MOH-dee-əs)

From English prefix **dis-,** with a negative meaning, + **commodious,** meaning "roomy."

troublesome; inconvenient; disadvantageous.

"When Peter finally found out that running away meant leaving the comforts of home and being able to afford only a **discommodi-**

ous one-room apartment and meals taken invariably in a greasy spoon, regret began to seep in and eventually overwhelm him."

Related words: **discommodiously** (DIS-kə-MOH-dee-əs-lee) *adverb*; **discommodiousness** (DIS-kə-MOH-dee-əs-nis) *noun*; **discommode** (DIS-kə-MOHD) *verb*.

discreet (di-SKREET)

From Middle English *discret*, meaning "circumspect, wise"; and Latin *discretus*, with the same meanings.

See also **discrete** for the difference in spelling and for the difference in meanings that have arisen in the many years since **discreet** and **discrete** became discrete English words.

1. circumspect; showing discernment or good judgment in speech and actions.

"My father always stressed the importance of the work he did for the government and the need for my being **discreet** in my speech, especially when people outside the family might be listening."

2. unostentatious; modest.

"The **discreet** jewelry she habitually wore never attracted attention, and few people even noticed it."

Related words: **discreetly** (di-SKREET-lee) *adverb*; **discreetness** (di-SKREET-nis) *noun*.

discrete (di-SKREET)

From the same Middle English and Latin sources as **discreet**.

You may wonder how English can have two words spelled so nearly alike yet have distinct meanings. From about the fourteenth century on, the intention was that there would be only one word. That the word soon was spelled in two different ways is not surprising because spelling had not yet become standardized, and **discreet** and **discrete** were going their merry ways.

When correct spelling grew to be considered rather important, in approximately the sixteenth century, men and women who wrote didactic spellers—spelling books whose main purpose was to teach—decided they would define the two words differently. They severed their meanings so each received a fair share, and the words were spelled approximately the way the words are spelled today.

distinct and discontinuous; detached from others.

"The challenging route to a million-dollar prize required that one answer fifteen **discrete** questions, some quite easy, a few extremely difficult."

See also **indiscrete.**

Related words: **discretely** (di-SKREET-lee) *adverb*; **discreteness** (di-SKREET-nis) *noun.*

discursive (di-SKUR-siv)
From Latin *discurrere*, meaning "to run to and fro."

1. digressive; chattering aimlessly.

"I might have paid more attention to the lecturer if she had been less **discursive** and better organized."

2. ratiocinative; moving ahead by reasoning and logic.

"All six lectures in the series proved splendidly **discursive** and easily absorbed by those who think logically."

Related words: **discursively** (di-SKUR-siv-lee) *adverb*; **discursiveness** (di-SKUR-siv-nis) and **discursion** (di-SKUR-zhən) *both nouns.*

disembodied (DIS-em-BOD-eed)
From English **dis-,** a prefix here meaning "apart," + **embody,** meaning "embrace."

of a spirit: divested of a body; separated from that in which it had been embodied.

"In the comedy the **disembodied** spirit of the man's first wife completely upsets his second marriage."

Related words: **disembody** (DIS-em-BOD-ee) *verb*; **disembodiment** (DIS-em-BOD-ee-mint) *noun.*

dishy (DISH-ee)
From British slang **dish,** meaning "an attractive woman," + **-y,** an adjectival suffix.

1. *British slang:* very attractive.

"He always chose to go to pubs that attracted a generous assortment of **dishy** girls."

2. *slang:* gossipy.

"Give her a **dishy** novel and a quiet room and you won't hear a word from her for hours."

disingenuous (DIS-in-JEN-yoo-əs)

From English **ingenuous,** meaning "naive."

Ingenuous used to be heard more often when we lived in simpler times, but as our history unfolds, we seem to have increased need for the meanings of **disingenuous.**

insincere; lacking in candor; hypocritically sincere.

"One had to be **disingenuous** rather than merely honest and hard-working to advance in that company."

Related words: **disingenuously** (DIS-in-JEN-yoo-əs-lee) *adverb*; **disingenuousness** (DIS-in-JEN-yoo-əs-nis) *noun*.

disinterested (dis-IN-tə-RES-tid)

From English **interested,** meaning "having a financial or other interest." Thus, a **disinterested** person has no financial or other interest in a company.

Even though many authorities suggest that **disinterested** also means "lacking interest," as in "I am disinterested in economics," be assured that nothing is gained from using the adjective in this misguided way. Indeed, nothing important will be lost from your writing if you use **disinterested** only in the sense given below—it might also be said your readers will understand you more easily if you never use **disinterested** in any other sense but the one now given.

unbiased; free of selfish motives.

"Many times he was accepted by attorneys for service on a jury because he appeared to be **disinterested** in the possible outcome of a trial."

Related words: **disinterestedly** (dis-IN-tə-RES-tid-lee) *adverb*; **disinterestedness** (dis-IN-tə-RES-tid-nis) *noun*.

disparate (DIS-pər-it)

From Latin *disparatus,* past participle of *disparare,* meaning "to segregate, divide."

dissimilar; essentially diverse in kind.

"They were a **disparate** group who found it difficult to cooperate with others toward what seemed to be a common goal."

Related words: **disparately** (DIS-pər-it-lee) *adverb*; **disparateness** (DIS-pər-it-nis) and **disparity** (di-SPA-ri-tee) *both nouns*.

dispirited (di-SPIR-i-tid)

From English verb **dispirit,** meaning "to deprive of spirit."

gloomy; discouraged; disheartened; dejected.

"I must report that my sister-in-law is still **dispirited,** many months after her son's untimely death."

Related words: **dispirit** (di-SPIR-it) *verb*; **dispiritedly** (di-SPIR-i-tid-lee) *adverb*; **dispiritedness** (di-SPIR-i-tid-nis) *noun*.

distingué (dee-stang-GAY)

From French *distingué*, past participle of *distinguer*, meaning "to distinguish."

distinguished; having an air of distinction.

"I always watched Dayton smoke his ivory-tipped cigarettes, which made him look so **distingué**; in my mind's eye, I could not hope to see myself ever looking that smart."

Related word: **distinguished** (di-STING-gwisht) *adjective*.

ditokous (DIT-ə-kəs)

From Greek *ditókos*, meaning "twin-bearing."

producing two young, or laying two eggs at a time.

"His rarest specimens were **ditokous,** but since one of the eggs in every clutch invariably broke, he almost never had any birds for sale."

ditsy (DIT-see)

Slang, origin unknown. Also given as **ditzy,** with the same pronunciation.

dizzy; eccentrically giddy, silly, inane.

"I have never become accustomed to all of Dora's **ditsy** ways, but my friends and I find her completely charming."

ditzy. *See* **ditsy.**

doctrinaire (DOK-trə-NAIR)

From French *doctrinaire*, meaning "dogmatic; pompous, sententious"; from Latin *doctrina*, meaning "doctrine." *See* **sententious.**

dogmatic; wedded to a particular philosophy and seeking to apply it in all circumstances.

"Crowley's **doctrinaire** attitudes in some areas lessened the true value of his scholarship."

Related words: **doctrinal** (DOK-trə-nl) *adjective;* doctrinally (DOK-trə-nə-lee) *adverb;* **doctrinality** (DOK-tri-NAL-i-tee) and **doctrine** (DOK-trin) *both nouns.*

doddering (DOD-ər-ing)

From Middle English *dadiren,* meaning "to tremble."

An adjective also given as **doddery** (DOD-ə-ree).

tottering; shaky or trembling as from age.

"Ferdinand, since I saw him last, has become a **doddering** old man who would be lost without his cane."

Related word: **dodder** (DOD-ər) *verb.*

dodgy (DOJ-ee)

From English infinitive **dodge,** meaning "to evade."

evasive; tricky; artful.

"Apparently because of his **dodgy** manner, no one trusts him, and trust is what he needs if he is to succeed in business."

Related words: **dodge** (doj) *verb;* **dodging** (DOJ-ing) and **dodger** (DOJ-ər) *both nouns.*

dolichocephalic (DOL-i-koh-sə-FAL-ik)

From Greek *dolichós,* meaning "long," + *kephalikós,* meaning "pertaining to the head."

Also given as **dolichocephalous** (DOL-i-koh-SEF-ə-ləs).

longheaded; having a skull whose width is about three-quarters of its length.

"Our anthropologists made careful measurements of all the aboriginal men and women we encountered and determined that the entire group clearly fell within the classification of **dolichocephalic** adults."

Related words: **dolichocephaly** (DOL-i-koh-SEF-ə-lee) and **dolichocephalism** (DOL-i-koh-SEF-ə-LIZ-əm) *both nouns.*

See **cephalic.**

donnish (DON-ish)

From English **don,** meaning "a tutor."

bookish; pedantic; pedantic in manner.

"He was put off by the **donnish** atmosphere and tried to avoid the company of his stuffy colleagues."

Related words: **donnishly** (DON-ish-lee) *adverb*; **donnishness** (DON-ish-nis) and **donnism** (DON-izm) *both nouns.*

dorky (DOR-kee)

Slang. Perhaps derived from vulgar slang **dork**, meaning "penis."

inept; foolishly stupid.

"You may think you have never heard anything more **dorky** in your life, but wait until you are treated to the full stupidity of my brother-in-law."

Related word: **dork** (dork) *noun.*

doughty (DOW-tee, rhymes with *loud he*)

From Middle English *douty*, meaning "worthy."

valiant; brave; formidable; steadfastly courageous.

"The marvelous old lady was fond of telling her grandchildren stories about their **doughty** father, who had served his country in two wars and been decorated twice for gallantry in action."

Related words: **doughtily** (DOW-ti-lee) *adverb*; **doughtiness** (DOW-ti-nis) *noun.*

dour (duur)

From Middle English, from Latin *durus*, meaning "harsh."

1. severe; hard; hardy.

"Sven had led a **dour** life trying to farm the rocky soil in the cruel northern climate."

2. stubborn; obstinate; hard to move; sullen.

"After Drew returned from his scouting mission beyond enemy lines, he became withdrawn, even **dour,** and remained that way, hardly ever speaking until long after the war was over."

Related words: **dourly** (DUUR-lee) *adverb*; **dourness** (DUUR-nis) *noun.*

Draconian (dray-KOH-nee-ən)

From Latin *Draco*, the name of a severe ancient Athenian jurist.

Also given as **draconic** and **Draconic** (both pronounced dray-KON-ik) and **draconian.**

1. characteristic of Draco or his harsh laws.

"The seventh century B.C. is the period we identify first with **Draconian** justice, a legal code notorious for its uncompromising criminal sentences."

2. rigorous; harsh; severe; cruel.

"Any law so **draconian** must surely be tested carefully before being applied, lest innocent or marginally guilty persons be punished unduly."

Related word: **Draconianism** (dray-KOH-nee-ən-izm) *noun.*

drossy (DRAW-see)

From Middle English *drosse,* from Old English *dros,* both meaning "dregs"; from English **dross,** meaning "scum or waste matter."

1. containing waste matter.

"The goldsmith was chagrined to find that the gold jewelry he recently bought had been stolen and was surely **drossy.**"

2. worthless; resembling waste matter.

"Reputable art auction houses are scrupulous about refusing to sponsor **drossy** collections, no matter how highly the public regards the collections."

Related words: **dross** (draws) and **drossiness** (DRAW-see-nis) *both nouns.*

droughty (DROW-tee)

From English **drought,** meaning "an extended dry spell."

Also given as **drouthy** (DROW-*th*ee).

arid, dry; deficient in rainfall.

"By the time the third year of **droughty** conditions had passed, the apple growers in Alfred's valley had sold their acreage and moved out."

Related words: **drought** (drowt) and **droughtiness** (DROWT-ee-nis) *both nouns.*

duplicitous (doo-PLIS-i-təs)

From English **duplicity,** meaning "deceit, double-dealing."

characterized by dishonesty or double-dealing.

"Our town was too small to enable an obviously **duplicitous** person to perform his shenanigans unnoticed."

Related words: **duplicity** (doo-PLIS-i-tee) *noun;* **duplicitously** (doo-PLIS-i-təs-lee) *adverb.*

duteous (DOO-tee-əs)

From English **duty,** meaning "obligation."

obedient; subservient; dutiful.

"The maid was at all times **duteous** and quiet while she was at work, but on her day off each week she seemed never silent."

Related words: **duteously** (DOO-tee-əs-lee) *adverb*; **duteousness** (DOO-tee-əs-nis) *noun*.

E

ebullient (i-BUUL-yənt)
From Latin *ebulliens,* present participle of infinitive *ebullire,* meaning "to bubble up."

1. highly enthusiastic; bubbling over with enthusiasm.

    "The entire country burst out in an **ebullient** celebration when World War II officially ended."

2. agitated; boiling; as if boiling.

    "When they reached the platform the department had built fifty yards from the top of the volcano, the temperature was so elevated that they were able to observe the **ebullient** lava for no more than a few minutes at a time."

    Related words: **ebullience** (i-BUUL-yəns) and **ebullition** (EB-ə-LISH-ən) *both nouns;* **ebulliently** (i-BUUL-yənt-lee) *adverb.*

eclectic (i-KLEK-tik)
From Greek *eklektikós,* meaning "selective."

heterogeneous, selecting from diverse doctrines, methods, and the like.

"They claimed that an **eclectic** approach offered a wider perspective than strict adherence to established methodology."

Related words: **eclectically** (i-KLEK-ti-klee) *adverb;* **eclecticism** (i-KLEK-tə-SIZ-əm) and **eclecticist** (i-KLEK-tə-sist) *both nouns.*

edacious (i-DAY-shəs)
From English noun **edacity,** from Latin *edacitas,* meaning "gluttony."

voracious; devoted to eating.

"We soon took to calling him **edacious** Eddy or hungry Eddy, but he never seemed to gain an ounce in weight."

edacity. *See* **edacious.**

edentulous (ee-DEN-chə-ləs)

From Latin *edentulus*, meaning "toothless."

Also given as **edentate** (ee-DEN-tayt).

toothless; having no teeth.

"The young social worker admitted that her textbooks had not prepared her for anything like the old hag's **edentulous** smile."

effable (EF-ə-bəl)

From former French *effable*, from Latin *effabilis*, meaning "capable of being expressed."

Effable is scarcely heard anymore, but it is currently hidden within the English word **ineffable,** meaning "indescribable or unspeakable": "She experienced an **ineffable** happiness that showed in her every action."

expressible; utterable.

"I was stunned to find her **effable** when she received the horrible news."

effete (i-FEET)

From Latin masculine *effetus*, meaning "exhausted"; Latin feminine *effeta*, meaning "exhausted from bearing young."

1. degenerate; decadent.

"His entire family was clearly **effete** after generations of profligate living on the great-grandfather's fortune."

2. enervated; exhausted; worn out; sterile.

"The great political party his father once represented was now seen as **effete,** incapable of mounting a vigorous campaign and losing election after election by increasing margins."

Related words: **effetely** (i-FEET-lee) *adverb*; **effeteness** (i-FEET-nis) *noun*.

efficacious (EF-i-KAY-shəs)

From Latin *efficax*, meaning "effective, capable."

of an object, instrument, etc.: having the strength to produce a desired effect.

"Human sweat is known for its inglorious but **efficacious** power of helping us achieve the impossible."

Related words: **efficaciously** (EF-i-KAY-shəs-lee) *adverb*; **efficaciousness** (EF-i-KAY-shəs-nis), **efficacy** (EF-i-kə-see), and **efficacity** (EF-i-KAS-i-tee) *all nouns*.

effulgent (i-FUL-jənt)

From Latin *effulgens*, present participle of infinitive *effulgere*, meaning "to shine out, blaze."

resplendent, radiant; shining forth brilliantly.

"The **effulgent** lake shimmered in the setting sun, hiding our children from view."

Related words: **effulgently** (i-FUL-jənt-lee) *adverb*; **effulgence** (i-FUL-jəns) *noun*.

effusive (i-FYOO-siv)

From English **effuse**, meaning "to pour out" + -*ive*, an adjectival suffix.

of emotions: irrepressible; unduly demonstrative.

"Eloise's parents were **effusive** in praise of their daughter's timorous fiancé, who stood before them in full anticipation of rejection."

Related words: **effusively** (i-FYOO-siv-lee) *adverb*; **effuse** (i-FYOOZ) *verb*; **effusiveness** (i-FYOO-siv-nis) and **effusion** (i-FYOO-zhən) *both nouns*.

egregious (i-GREE-jəs)

From Latin adjective *egregius*, meaning "illustrious"; from *e-*, meaning "outside," + *grex*, meaning "flock," + -*ius*, an adjectival suffix.

A word suggesting beautifully that a black sheep always stands out in a flock of snow-white creatures.

conspicuously bad in a flagrant way.

"He grumbled that I was an **egregious** liar, but I felt sure he had no real evidence of my misdeeds."

Related words: **egregiously** (i-GREE-jəs-lee) *adverb*; **egregiousness** (i-GREE-jəs-nis) *noun*.

eldritch (EL-drich)

From Middle English *elfriche*, meaning "fairyland."

spooky, weird, eerie; hideous.

"That night I searched for him in the **eldritch** town, with bats, cats, and indistinct figures lurking in the shadows."

eleemosynary (EL-ə-MOS-ə-NER-ee)
From Middle Latin *eleemosynarius,* meaning "compassionate."

1. supported by charity or dependent on it.

"There is good reason to treat **eleemosynary** institutions as tax-exempt entities as long as they can show their funds are mostly dependent on charitable work."

2. gratuitous; charitable in purpose.

"Together, the board members of the **eleemosynary** organization managed to contribute enough money to fund operation of the children's athletic teams for the entire season."

emeritus (i-MER-i-təs)
From Latin *emeritus,* meaning "having fully earned"; past participle of *emerere,* meaning "to deserve, earn fully."

One of the most interesting aspects of the term **emeritus** is that it has a second meaning, that of "being worn out."

Everyone who has firsthand acquaintance with **emeritus** professors or with **emerita** (feminine) professors knows that retired scholars neither fade away nor wear out. More likely, they collapse from fatigue and boredom.

By contrast, those who receive honorary degrees—because they have never taught a day in their lives but have given honor to the institution, or lots of money—leave immediately after the ceremony completely rested, to tee up at an exclusive golf course.

honorably retired from active service and with the same title held before retirement.

"Two of our oldest department heads this year will be given **emeritus** titles in recognition of their distinguished careers as teachers and scholars."

Related word: **emerita** (i-MER-i-tə) *adjective.*

emollient (i-MOL-yənt)
From Latin *emolliens,* meaning "softening up," present participle of *emollire,* meaning "to soften."

Not to be confused with the noun **emolument** (i-MOL-yə-mənt), "a fee or other money payment for services rendered."

soothing; having the power of softening, especially the skin.

"Mr. Cowperthwaite made his fortune by selling a line of patent medicines, beginning with **emollient** salves for skin overexposed to sun and wind."

Related word: **emollience** (i-MOL-yəns) *noun*.

emolument. *See* **emollient.**

emulous (EM-yə-ləs)

From Latin *aemulus*, meaning "rivaling; jealous."

desirous of rivaling or surpassing.

"Girls, **emulous** of their older sisters, cannot wait to begin using lipstick and eye makeup in preparation for important dates."

Related words: **emulously** (EM-yə-ləs-lee) *adverb*; **emulate** (EM-yə-LAYT) *verb*; **emulative** (EM-yə-LAY-tiv) *adjective*; **emulousness** (EM-yə-ləs-nis) *noun*.

emunctory (i-MUNGK-tə-ree)

From Modern Latin *emunctorius*, meaning "excretory," from Latin *emungere*, meaning "to wipe the nose."

excretory; of the blowing of the nose.

"During the season of winter colds, our concerts were punctuated with annoying **emunctory** activity."

encomiastic (en-KOH-mee-AS-tik)

From Greek *enkomiastés*, from *enkómion*, meaning "a eulogy," + *-astes*, a suffix meaning "one who (delivers)."

eulogistic; laudatory, commendatory.

"The **encomiastic** master of ceremonies is unsurpassed at introducing speakers, missing not a single beat in delivering anything desired, from a few ounces of faint praise to wild exaggeration."

Related words: **encomium** (en-KOH-mee-əm) *noun*; **encomiastically** (en-KOH-mee-AS-ti-kal-ee) *adverb*.

enervated (EN-ər-VAY-tid)

From Latin *enervatus*, meaning "weakened," past participle of *enervare*, "to weaken; unman."

Also given as the adjectives **enervate** (i-NUR-vit) and **enervative** (EN-ər-VAY-tiv), with the same meanings.

languid; without vigor or strength; effeminate.

"The **enervated** senior counsel lacks the determination needed to make a vigorous case in defense of the accused."

Related words: **enervation** (EN-ər-VAY-shən) and **enervator** (EN-ər-VAY-tər) *both nouns.*

entomophagous (EN-tə-MOF-ə-gəs)

From English **entomo-,** a combining form meaning "insect," + **-phagous,** a combining form meaning "eating or feeding on."

insectivorous; insect eating.

"For twelve years he has been happily dissecting the innards of **entomophagous** beetles in hope of identifying all their prey."

ephemeral (i-FEM-ər-əl)

From Greek *ephémeros,* meaning "lasting only for a day."

Also given as **ephemerous** (i-FEM-ər-əs).

1. of reputation, popularity, institutions, and the like: transitory; short-lived.

"Little did they know it, but the democracy they extolled was **ephemeral,** built not on a secure footing but in conformity with a poorly understood model."

2. of insects or anything else deemed to be short-lived: lasting only a day or the equivalent.

"When all the dot.coms were in their heyday, nobody really knew whether any of them would prove to be more than **ephemeral.**"

Related words: **ephemerally** (i-FEM-ər-əl-ee) *adverb;* **ephemeralness** (i-FEM-ər-əl-nis), **ephemera** (i-FEM-ər-ə), **ephemerality** (i-FEM-ə-RAL-i-tee), **ephemeron** (i-FEM-ə-RON), plural **ephemera** (i-FEM-ə-rə), *all nouns.*

It is interesting to note that the singular **ephemeron,** in the sense of "anything ephemeral," is rarely heard, while the plural **ephemera** in the sense of "items intended to be used for a short time," is much more common. And what does that say about our civilization?

epicene (EP-i-SEEN)

From Latin *epicoenus,* meaning "of both genders," from Greek *epíkoinos,* meaning "common to many."

1. possessing characteristics of both sexes.

"Now, in our haste to speak and write of so-called genderless every-things, we are treated to **epicene** fashions, unisex barber shops, and his-and-her cigar clubs."

2. feeble; flaccid.

"Fans of his rip-roaring adventure novels are surprised by his **epicene** handshake."

3. effeminate.

"We soon found that our **epicene** new department head was a severe person, brooking no foolishness from his subordinates."

Related word: **epicenism** (EP-i-SEEN-iz-əm) *noun.*

epidemic. *See* **pandemic.**

epistolary (i-PIS-tə-LER-ee)

From Latin *epistolaris,* meaning "belonging to a letter."

Also given as **epistolic** (EP-ə-STOL-ik) and as **epistolical** (EP-ə-STOL-i-kəl).

carried on or contained in letters.

"The **epistolary** novel can be an exciting form when writers reveal insights they understand and feel."

Related words: **epistle** (i-PIS-əl), **epistoler** (i-PIS-tl-ər), **epistolist** (i-PIS-tə-list), and **epistler** (i-PIS-lər) *all nouns;* **epistolize** (i-PIS-tl-īz) *verb.*

eponymous (ə-PON-ə-məs)

From Greek epónymos, meaning "giving name (to)."

giving one's name to a people, place, etc.

"Brut, said to have been a grandson of Aeneas, is generally consid-ered the **eponymous** progenitor of Britain."

Related words: **eponym** (EP-ə-nim) and **eponymy** (ə-PON-ə-mee) *both nouns.*

eristic (e-RIS-tik)

From Greek *eristikós,* "wrangling."

Also given as **eristical** (e-RIS-ti-kəl).

controversial; pertaining to controversy or disputation.

"Adler's philosophy classes consisted of thirteen weeks of **eristic** exercises, undeniably a tribute to Eris, the ancient Greek god-

dess of discord, but ostensibly intended to teach the art of disputation."

Related word: **eristically** (er-IS-ti-kə-lee).

eructative (i-RUK-tə-tiv)

From Latin *eructatus*, meaning "thrown up"; from infinitive *eructare*,
meaning "to belch, emit."

1. of a person: given to belching or vomiting.

"By the time the attending physicians had completed their analysis,
Timothy was in danger of succumbing to a continuous state of
eructative activity."

2. of a volcano: given to belching matter.

"Last night, I was given the privilege of seeing two hours of rough
footage of **eructative** volcanoes."

Related words: **eruct** (i-RUKT) and **eructate** (i-RUK-tayt) *both
verbs*; **eructation** (i-ruk-TAY-shən) *noun*.

esculent (ES-kyə-lənt)

From Latin *esculentus*, meaning "edible, tasty"; from *esca*, meaning
"food, tidbits."

edible, eatable; suitable as food.

"Many beginners were surprised to learn how many **esculent** plants
could be found growing as weeds."

esurient (i-SUUR-ee-ənt)

From Latin *esuriens*, meaning "hungering," present participle of
infinitive *esurire*, meaning "to be hungry for, to hunger."

greedy; hungry.

"Some **esurient** young lawyers are willing to take any case that
comes their way but soon enough commit their time only to cases
that promise big fees."

evanescent (EV-ə-NES-ənt)

From Latin *evanescens*, present participle of verb *evanescere*, meaning
"to vanish."

fleeting; fading away or quickly vanishing.

"As the days of summer went on, Joe saw his **evanescent** chances of
victory gradually disappearing."

Related words: **evanesce** (EV-ə-NES) *verb*; **evanescence** (EV-ə-NES-əns) *noun;* **evanescible** (EV-ə-NES-i-bəl) *adjective;* **evanescently** (EV-ə-NES-ənt-lee) *adverb.*

excrementitious (EK-skrə-men-TISH-əs)

From English **excrement,** meaning "feces," + **-itious,** an adjectival suffix; from Latin *excrementum,* meaning "waste matter."

of the nature of excrement; like waste matter.

"Almost all insects are seen to emit drops of **excrementitious** matter each time they ingest food."

Related words: **excrete** (ik-SKREET) *verb;* **excrement** (EK-skrə-mənt), **excreta** (ik-SKREE-tə), and **excretion** (ik-SKREE-shən) *all nouns;* **excrementous** (EK-skrə-MEN-təs) and **excretal** (ik-SKREE-təl) *both adjectives;* **excrementitiously** (EK-skrə-men-TISH-əs-lee) and **excrementally** (EK-skrə-MEN-tə-lee) *both adverbs.*

excrescent (ik-SKRES-ənt)

From Latin *excrescens,* present participle of *excrescere,* meaning "to grow, rise up."

growing abnormally out of something else.

"The emergency room at our hospital is busy night and day, treating patients, sewing wounds, and occasionally arranging for consultations on **excrescent** growths."

Related words: **excrescently** (ik-SKRES-ənt-lee) *adverb;* **excrescence** (ik-SKRES-əns) and **excrescency** (ik-SKRES-ən-see) *both nouns.*

exculpatory (ik-SKUL-pə-TOR-ee)

From English **exculpate,** meaning "free from blame"; from Medieval Latin infinitive *exculpare,* meaning "to declare guiltless."

of evidence, argument, etc.: tending to clear from blame.

"My **exculpatory** deposition, along with the testimony of several character witnesses, appeared to help the defendant's case somewhat."

Related words: **exculpate** (EK-skul-PAYT) *verb;* **exculpable** (ik-SKUL-pə-bəl) *adjective;* **exculpation** (IK-skul-PAY-shən) *noun.*

execrable (EK-si-krə-bəl)

From Middle English *execrable* from Latin *execrabilis,* meaning "accursed, detestable; deadly."

1. of persons and things: abominable; deserving to be cursed.

   "In our little town, this **execrable** pedophile is going to have a difficult time finding a disinterested jury and an experienced lawyer to defend him."

2. bad beyond description.

   "Any soprano so tuneless, so limited in range, can expect to be attacked in the press and even characterized as **execrable**."

   Related words: **execrably** (EK-si-krə-blee) and **execratively** (EK-si-KRAY-tiv-lee) *both adverbs*; **execration** (EK-si-KRAY-shən) and **execrableness** (EK-si-krə-bəl-nis) *both nouns*; **execrate** (EK-si-KRAYT) *verb*; **execrative** (EK-si-KRAY-tiv) and **execratory** (EK-si-krə-TOR-ee) *both adjectives*.

exegetic (EK-si-JET-ik)
From Greek *exegetikós*, meaning "to interpret, guide, or lead."

Also given in English as the adjective **exegetical** (EK-si-JET-ik-əl).

interpretive: explanatory.

   "The minister's feeble attempts to provide an **exegetic** framework for the sermon served only to further complicate matters."

   Related words: **exegetically** (EK-si-JET-ik-ə-lee) *adverb*; **exegesis** (EK-si-JEE-səs), **exegete** (EK-si-JEET), and **exegetist** (EK-si-JET-ist) *all nouns*.

exiguous (ig-ZIG-yoo-əs)
From Latin *exiguus*, meaning "meager, small."

scanty; small; meager; slender; diminutive.

   "On his **exiguous** income, the couple were able to get along somehow and even support a small child."

   Related words: **exiguously** (ig-ZIG-yoo-əs-lee) *adverb*; **exiguity** (EK-si-GYOO-i-tee) and **exiguousness** (ek-ZIG-yoo-əs-nis) *both nouns*.

expiable (EK-spee-ə-bəl)
From Late Latin *expiabilis*, meaning "capable of being atoned"; from the Latin infinitive *expiare*, meaning "to make satisfaction."

capable of expiating; atoning for; making amends.

   "Business sins may be **expiable** merely by confessing, but felonious crimes frequently must be paid for in considerable time spent behind bars."

Related words: **expiate** (EK-spee-AYT) *verb;* **expiator** (EK-spee-AY-tor) and **expiation** (EK-spee-AY-shən) *both nouns;* **expiational** (EK-spee-AY-shən-əl) and **expiatory** (EK-spee-ə-TOR-ee) *both adjectives.*

expostulatory (ik-SPOS-chə-lə-TOR-ee)

From English **expostulate,** meaning "remonstrate"; from Latin *expostulatus,* past participle of infinitive *expostulare,* meaning "to demand urgently; protest, complain of."

Expostulatory is also given as the adjective **expostulative** (ik-SPOS-chə-LAY-tiv).

by way of remonstrance; conveying or characterized by expostulation.

"Mary tried again to write an earnest **expostulatory** letter to the ecclesiastical court but failed to complete it and soon abandoned her quest for adjudication."

Related words: **expostulatingly** (ik-SPOS-chə-LAY-ting-lee) *adverb;* **expostulator** (ik-SPOS-chə-LAY-tər) and **expostulation** (ik-SPOS-chə-LAY-shən) *both nouns.*

expugnable (ek-SPYOO-nə-bəl)

From Latin *expugnabilis,* meaning "capable of being taken by storm," from *ex-,* a prefix meaning "thoroughly," + *pugnare,* meaning "to fight."

Considered by some an archaic word, nevertheless included here because it is so attractive.

While most of us know the word **impugn,** meaning "to challenge someone for speaking or acting falsely" and its related word **impugnable,** we scarcely hear of **expugnable.** So we regularly **impugn** someone's motives, but we almost never consider anything **expugnable.** Might you say we are more and more suspicious but less and less eager for a fight?

conquerable; that may be overcome.

"I know my supervisor's position on this matter is **expugnable,** but I also know he and his associates will never forgive me for being correct."

extra-virgin (EK-strə-VUR-jin)

A verbal curiosity, included here to have some fun. The adjective derives of course from the English **extra** and **virgin.** It also, of course, lacks direct connection to the meanings of these two words. It does, however, relate to **virgin**—pure as the driven snow. And

extra appears to be an instance of the hyperbole that advertising geniuses regularly exploit.

Virgin oil actually is the oil obtained, usually from olives, by the first pressing of the fruit without application of heat. And what does that have to do with virginity, the chaste condition that human females and other females generally start out life with? Could the use of pressure in the **extra-virgin** process without applying heat have something to with the flavor of the oil? Or is there some conditional mode of human behavior associated with first-time oil-extraction or first-time sex? Whatever the advantage of this mysterious first-time pressing of oil from olives, we are inevitably confronted with the implication that this is no ordinary oil extraction.

"Remember, an olive oil may be **extra-virgin,** in the sense of even more pure than merely virginal, and usually thought of as better than expected."

It is not some additional pressure exerted on unmarried women.

F

fabular (FAB-yə-lər)

> From Latin *fabularis*, meaning "fabular," from *fabula*, meaning "story, fable, etc." *See also* **fabulous.**

of the nature of a fable; fabulous.

> "Although we knew most of his stories were predominantly **fabular,** they held especial fascination for us."

> Related words: **fabulist** (FAB-yə-list) *noun;* **fabled** (FAY-bəld) *adjective.*

fabulous (FAB-yə-ləs)

> From Latin *fabulosus,* meaning "legendary"; see **fabular.**

1. incredible: difficult to believe.

> "The **fabulous** feats the freshman team achieved brought them a collection of gold medals that surpassed those of any other team."

2. imaginary, entirely mythical: told in fables.

> "As a child I never tired of reading accounts of the **fabulous** achievements of the Martian warriors, of the depredations of terrible dragons, and of the havoc wrought by fire-breathing monsters."

> Related words: **fabulously** (FAB-yə-ləs-lee) *adverb;* **fabulousness** (FAB-yə-ləs-nis) *noun.*

facetious (fə-SEE-shəs)

> From French *facétieux,* meaning "facetious, mischievous"; from Latin plural *facetiae,* meaning "wit, clever talk"; from *facetus,* meaning "witty, clever."

1. not intended to be taken seriously.

"Walter's annoying habit of injecting **facetious** remarks into otherwise serious conversations finally got him into real trouble with his fiancée's father and threatened to delay his marriage indefinitely."

2. jocular: lacking serious purpose.

"When I first met Brenda in school, I saw her as a **facetious** scholar, interested only in enjoying her allotted four years and seriously intent on learning nothing."

Related words: **facetiously** (fə-SEE-shəs-lee) *adverb*; **facetiousness** (fə-SEE-shəs-nis) *noun*.

factious (FAK-shəs)
From Latin *factiosus*, meaning "contentious, quarrelsome, dissentious."

1. given to discord or dissension.

"Strong leadership does not tolerate **factious** divisiveness, which robs an organization of its effectiveness."

2. proceeding from factional interest.

"Not much happened in most of our meetings, steeped as they were in **factious** quarrels that ended in hopeless deadlocks."

Related words: **factiously** (FAK-shəs-lee) *adverb*; **factiousness** (FAK-shəs-nis), **faction** (FAK-shən), **factoid** (FAK-toid) *all nouns*; **factional** (FAK-shə-nl) *adjective*.

factitious (fak-TISH-əs)
From Latin *facticius*, meaning "artificial."

artificial; unspontaneous; manufactured.

"I'm tired of **factitious** sitcoms, with their canned laughter and applause, with their pretended nudity, and their absence of entertainment value."

Related words: **factitiously** (fak-TISH-əs-lee) *adverb*; **factitiousness** (fak-TISH-əs-nis) *noun*.

falcate (FAL-kayt)
From Latin *falcatus*, meaning "sickle shaped."

Also given as **falciform** (FAL-sə-FORM) and as **falcated** (FAL-kay-tid).

hooked; curved like a sickle.

"The eagle has a **falcate** beak, which enables the bird to pull apart its prey while sailing high in the sky."

Related words: **falx** (falks) and **falcon** (FAWL-kən) *both nouns*; **falcial** (FAL-shəl) *adjective*.

Falstaffian (fawl-STAF-ee-ən)

From the name of **Sir John Falstaff,** the fat, self-indulgent, and jovial braggart of Shakespeare's *The Merry Wives of Windsor* and *Henry IV*, Parts 1 and 2.

having the qualities of Falstaff; bawdy-humored, rascally, and bragging.

"By the time Barry reached adulthood, he had eaten and drunk his way into becoming a **Falstaffian** figure and was scarcely regarded seriously by his contemporaries."

fantabulous (fan-TAB-yə-ləs)

An English slang blend of **fantastic + fabulous.**

of almost incredible excellence.

"Joe, Mickey, and the Babe were three of a handful of **fantabulous** sluggers who established and sustained the Yankee mystique of the century past."

farraginous (fə-RAJ-ə-nəs)

From Latin noun *farrago,* meaning "a hodgepodge; mash, medley of grains," taken into English + English suffix *-ous,* meaning "full of."

heterogeneous; miscellaneous.

"What we finally had on hand after so many hours of aimless library research and almost aimless writing was a **farraginous** aggregation of stray information, much of it useless for our project."

Related word: **farrago** (fə-RAH-goh) *noun.*

fastuous (FAS-choo-əs)

From Latin *fastuosus,* from *fastus,* meaning "haughtiness, arrogance."

haughty, arrogant; pretentious, ostentatious.

"From the moment he took office, he appeared to be transformed from the trustworthy good old boy we thought we had elected into a **fastuous** windbag."

Related word: **fastuously** (FAS-choo-əs-lee) *adverb.*

fatidic (fay-TID-ik)

From Latin *fatidicus,* meaning "prophetic."

Also given as **fatidical** (fay-TID-ik-əl).

prophetic.

"Jean doesn't seem to mind that her **fatidic** pronouncements invariably prove incorrect."

Related word: **fatidically** (fay-TID-i-kə-lee) *adverb*.

fatigable (FAT-i-gə-bəl)
From Latin *fatigabilis*, from infinitive *fatigare*, meaning "to tire."

Another of those words that are better known in the negative, **indefatigable** (in-di-FAT-i-gə-bəl), than in the positive, **fatigable**. Perhaps, whether true or not, an indication of the backbone inherent in all English speakers: we do not tire easily. At any rate we do have the word **fatigable**, also given as **fatiguable** (fə-TEEG-ə-bəl) and as **fatigued** (fə-TEEGD).

subject to fatigue; easily tired.

"Less than halfway through the arduous climb, many of the **fatigable** group acknowledged that they had not prepared adequately for the expedition."

Related words: **fatigableness** (FAT-i-gə-bəl-nis) and **fatigability** (FAT-i-gə-BIL-ə-tee) *both nouns*; **fatigueless** (fə-TEEG-lis) *adjective*; **fatiguingly** (fə-TEEG-ing-lee) *adverb*.

fatuous (FACH-oo-əs)
From Latin *fatuus*, meaning "foolish, silly, insipid."

Also given as **fatuitous** (fə-TOO-i-təs).

of persons or their actions: foolish, silly, inane, especially in a complacent manner.

"Herbert's **fatuous** disregard for his wife's feelings was entirely reprehensible in one who professed to be a decent and honorable man."

Related words: **fatuously** (FACH-oo-əs-lee) *adverb*; **fatuity** (fə-TOO-i-tee) and **fatuousness** (FACH-oo-əs-nis) *both nouns*.

favonian (fə-VOH-nee-ən)
From Latin *Favonianus*, "the west wind"; from the name *Favonius*, an ancient Roman personification of the west wind; from infinitive *favere*, meaning "to favor, befriend, support."

propitious; pertaining to the west wind, therefore mild or favorable.

"The preacher went about within his church, opening all the windows in hope, he said, of attracting **favonian** zephyrs laden with the aromas of spring."

febrifacient (FEB-rə-FAY-shənt)

> From Latin *febris*, meaning "fever," + *-facient*, a combining form meaning "making." From present participle of *facere*, meaning "to make," thus "fever-making."

> Also given as **febriferous** (fi-BRIF-ər-əs).

> fever-producing.

>> "My grandfather believed a strong shot of scotch, in which he saw **febrifacient** qualities, plus a protracted spell in bed did more to induce sweating and cure sickness than all the medicines known to man."

>> Related words: **febricity** (fi-BRIS-i-tee) *noun;* **febrific** (fi-BRIF-ik), **febrifugal** (fi-BRIF-yə-gəl), and **febrile** (FEB-rəl) *all adjectives;* **febrifuge** (FEB-rə-FYOOJ) *adjective* and *noun.*

febriferous. *See* **febrifacient.**

febrific. *See* **febrifacient.**

febrile. *See* **febrifacient.**

fecaloid (FE-kə-LOYD)

> From English **feces,** meaning "excrement," + **-oid,** an adjectival suffix meaning "like."

> resembling feces.

>> "The repulsive vomit he expelled was **fecaloid** in odor and made us all gag."

feckless (FEK-lis)

> From Scottish and northern English **feck,** meaning "effect," + **-less,** an adjectival suffix meaning "without," thus "without effect."

> Which makes one wonder whether there also is a *feckful* and, as it turns out, there once was a *feckful* in Scottish and in the English spoken in England's north. It meant "efficient, powerful." Apparently, nothing beats being full of feck.

> of people: ineffective, incompetent; weak, helpless; indifferent, lazy, irresponsible.

>> "The family blamed the loss of their fortune on bad luck and the dishonesty of others, but the truth is they were **feckless** and frittered it away."

>> Related words: **fecklessly** (FEK-lis-lee) *adverb;* **fecklessness** (FEK-lis-nis) *noun.*

feculent (FEK-yə-lənt)

From Latin *faeculentus*, meaning "full of dregs"; from Latin *faeces*, singular *faex*, meaning "grounds, sediment; feces."

foul, turbid; polluted with feces.

"Obviously, the **feculent** water was not fit to drink, nor would it be drunk until a drenching rain had a chance to clarify the stream."

Related words: **fecula** (FEK-yə-lə) and **feculence** (FEK-yə-ləns) *both nouns.*

fecund (FEE-kuund)

From Latin *fecundus*, meaning "fruitful."

1. of animals, the earth, etc.: capable of reproduction, capable of abundant growth.

"After several years of composting, the sod had become so **fecund** that we were able to grow enough vegetables for our own family and several others."

2. intellectually creative.

"Our century has not produced all the musical geniuses we may have wanted, but it still could be considered **fecund** even without Bach, Beethoven, or Brahms."

Related words: **fecundity** (fi-KUN-di-tee) and **fecundation** (FEE-kun-DAY-shən) *both nouns;* **fecundatory** (fi-KUN-də-TOR-ee) *adjective;* **fecundate** (FEE-kən-DAYT) *verb.*

feisty (FĪ-stee)

From American slang; from **feist,** meaning "a mutt," + **-y,** a suffix meaning "like a (something)."

aggressive; excitable; touchy; troublesome.

"My wife's grandfather was a **feisty** old man who could deal with anyone who tried to take advantage of him."

Related words: **feist** (fīst) *noun;* **feistily** (FĪST-ə-lee) *adverb;* **feistiness** (FĪST-ee-nis) *noun.*

fell (fel)

From Middle English *fel,* meaning "savage"; from Old French *felon,* meaning "wicked."

1. of animals and people: cruel, ruthless; dreadful.

"They exhibited **fell** ferocity toward those they considered their enemies and killed them in great numbers."

2. of poison: deadly, destructive.

"Scientists agreed that **fell** poisons had been administered by the mass murderer, who had to have been someone with access to such materials."

Related words: **felly** (FEL-ee) *adverb*; **fellness** (FEL-nis) *noun.*

fenestrated (FEN-ə-STRAY-tid)

From Latin *fenestratus,* meaning "equipped with windows," from *fenestra,* meaning "window."

Fenestrated is also given as the adjective **fenestrate** (fə-NES-trayt).

having windows.

"By the time Western homes were adequately **fenestrated,** windows were expected to do much more for the occupants than provide portholes for shooting arrows at marauders."

Related words: **fenestra** (fi-NES-trə) and **fenestration** (FEN-ə-STRAY-shən) *both nouns.*

feral (FER-əl)

From Medieval Latin *feralis,* meaning "wild, bestial"; from Latin *fera,* meaning "wild beast."

1. of an animal or plant: wild, undomesticated.

"The gamekeeper testified he was set upon by a pack of **feral** hounds and had no other means of self-defense but his rifle and a limited number of shells."

2. of a human: resembling a wild beast; brutal, savage.

"Crusoe had no way of knowing for certain whether the **feral** men and women he came upon were cannibals."

ferruginous (fə-ROO-jə-nəs)

From Latin *ferrugineus,* meaning "color of rust, dark," from *ferrum,* meaning "iron."

1. reddish-brown: resembling the color of iron rust.

"The ditsy interior decorator unfortunately chose **ferruginous** wallpaper to decorate the steel magnate's dining room."

2. relating to or containing iron.

"A pocket compass is of little use when one is hiking near cliffs containing **ferruginous** ores."

fescennine (FES-ə-NĪN)

From Latin *Fescenninus*, meaning "a ribald song"; also meaning "pertaining to *Fescennia*," an Etrurian town famous for its jeering dialogues in verse.

licentious, obscene, scurrilous.

"The best man's **fescennine** speech might have been more appropriate at a stag party than at the wedding dinner."

festinate (FES-tə-NAYT)

From Latin *festinatus*, meaning "hasty, hurried"; past participle of infinitive *festinare*, meaning "to hurry; hasten."

hasty, hurried.

"Her **festinate** packing of their three big suitcases made for much jollity when all the contents spilled across the table of the customs officer."

Related words: **festinately** (FES-tə-NAYT-lee) *adverb*; **festination** (FES-tə-NAY-shən) *noun*.

fetid (FET-id)

From Latin *fetidus*, meaning "stinking," from infinitive *fetere*, meaning "to have an offensive smell."

stinking; having an offensive smell.

"Secaucus, a New Jersey town that once was the center of pig breeding in metropolitan New York, was so well known for its **fetid** odor that pig farming there had to be made illegal."

Related words: **fetidly** (FET-id-lee) *adverb*; **fetidness** (FET-id-nis) and **fetidity** (fe-TID-i-tee) *both nouns*.

fictile (FIK-tl)

From Latin *fictilis*, meaning "earthen, moldable"; from past participle of *fingere*, meaning "to shape or fashion."

Which tells us metaphorically that **fiction**—unlike the book you are now reading—is molded of earth by artists. But solely metaphorically. *See* **fictitious**.

1. capable of being made of earth by a potter.

"Ancient battles and love affairs lent themselves to exploitation in permanent **fictile** creativity by the great artisans then at work."

2. of or pertaining to the manufacture of pottery.

"For unknown reasons the **fictile** craft flourished in Ohio early in the twentieth century."

fictional. *See* **fictitious.**

fictitious (fik-TISH-əs)

From Latin *ficticius*, meaning "artificial"; from *fictus*, past participle of *fingere*, meaning "to form, shape."

Observe that **fictitious** is sometimes given the meaning of **fictional**, as shown in the second definition below, but **fictional** is preferable in that sense, since it is generally taken as more restricted in meaning.

1. false; created for the purpose of concealment.

"As part of his plan for evading the law, Stephen adopted a **fictitious** name and identity."

2. fictional; imaginary; created by the imagination.

"A popular hero of the young in my day was Superman, a **fictitious** *Übermensch*, for whom no hardship was insuperable."

Better to have written "**fictional** *Übermensch* . . ."

Related words: **fictitiously** (fik-TISH-əs-lee) *adverb*; **fictitiousness** (fik-TISH-əs-nis) *noun*; **fictionalize** (FIK-shə-nl-ɪz) *verb*.

filose (FĪ-lohs)

From Latin *filum*, "a thread," + *-ose*, an adjectival suffix meaning "like."

Also given as **filiform** (FIL-ə-FORM), as in "The cardiac surgeon had the unenviable job of cutting away all the flesh around a **filiform** vein without abrading it."

threadlike; having a threadlike structure.

"On close examination I found the insect's **filose** antennae not quite broken through but clearly functioning imperfectly."

finicky (FIN-i-kee)

Of unknown origin, although several sources have been suggested. All of them seem to converge on the old reliable adjective **fine.**

Finicky is also given as **finical** (FIN-i-kəl).

fussy; inordinately fastidious; hard to please.

"It was not so much that she was **finicky** when ordering in a restaurant and tried the patience of waiters, but that she seemingly took forever to make up her mind and just moments to change it again."

Related word: **finick** (FIN-ik) *verb*.

fissile (FIS-əl)

From Latin *fissilis*, meaning "easy to split," a term now heard mainly in connection with nuclear physics, but formerly with log splitting.

cleavable; capable of being divided or split into parts.

"Care was taken to make sure sufficient **fissile** material would be stored in warehouses and available at the time planned for explosion of the early nuclear bombs."

Related words: **fission** (FISH-ən) and **fissionability** (FISH-ən-ə-BIL-i-tee) *both nouns*; **fissionable** (FISH-ə-nə-bəl) *adjective*.

flaccid (FLAK-sid)

From Latin *flaccidus*, meaning "flabby, feeble"; from infinitive *flaccere*, meaning "to flag, lose heart."

1. not firm; lacking normal firmness.

"Weeks of bed rest had robbed his body of its vitality, and the nurses knew his **flaccid** muscles would require careful treatment and exercise."

2. weak; lacking vigor or force.

"The **flaccid** paragraphs he turned in were not at all characteristic of the strong prose style to which we had been accustomed."

Related words: **flaccidly** (FLAK-sid-lee) *adverb*; **flaccidity** (flak-SID-i-tee) and **flaccidness** (FLAK-sid-nis) *both nouns*.

flagitious (flə-JISH-əs)

From Latin *flagitiosus*, meaning "shameful crime"; also "disgraceful, profligate."

We must understand that the Romans did not always agree on what was considered *flagitiosus*.

1. of people or their actions: shamefully wicked, extraordinarily criminal.

"Is it possible that the definition of a **flagitious** criminal has been weakened in the past century, which saw slaughter of ethnic groups numbering in the millions?"

2. of crime: villainous, infamous; heinous, flagrant.

"The mayor gleefully announced that the number of **flagitious** crimes had fallen 10 percent in the past year, but we wondered how many actual crimes in all were reported."

Related words: **flagitiously** (flə-JISH-əs-lee) *adverb*; **flagitiousness** (flə-JISH-əs-nis) *noun*.

flannelmouthed (FLAN-l-MOU*TH*D)

A contemptuous term from American **flannel**, "a soft fabric," + **mouth + -ed**, an adjectival suffix.

1. loudmouthed; boastful.

"That double-talking **flannelmouthed** neighbor of mine is embarrassing as well as boring."

2. deceptive in speech.

"His **flannelmouthed** responses to our forthright questions cause him to appear evasive and certainly shed no light on the problems we face."

Related words: **flannelmouth** (FLAN-l-MOUTH) *noun*; **flannelly** (FLAN-l-ee) *adjective*.

flatulent (FLACH-ə-lənt)

From Modern Latin *flatulentus*, meaning "gassy," from *flatus*, "a blowing," + *-ulent*, an adjectival suffix meaning "full of."

Latin, always interesting, also defines *flatulentus* as "arrogance." See what English has done to **flatulent**.

1. of a disease: generating gas in the intestinal tract.

"Her condition was often accompanied by **flatulent** episodes for which her physician's prescriptions did little good."

2. of a person: suffering an excess of such gas.

"Edmund, embarrassed by his obviously **flatulent** condition, almost never attended dinner parties in those days."

3. windy, pretentious; pompous, turgid.

"He was often taken to task by literary critics for his **flatulent** style, so loved by some writers."

See also **luculent** for a change of pace.

Related words: **flatus** (FLAY-təs), **flatulence** (FLACH-ə-ləns), and **flatulency** (FLACH-ə-lən-see) *all nouns*; **flatulently** (FLACH-ə-lənt-lee) *adverb*.

flavescent (flə-VES-ənt)

From Latin *flavescens*, present participle of infinitive *flavescere*, meaning "to become yellow," from *flavens* "yellow, golden."

yellowish; turning pale yellow.

"Alphonse finally achieved his goal of developing a distinctively **flavescent** hibiscus."

flexuous (FLEK-shoo-əs)

From Latin *flexuosus*, meaning "winding, full of curves"; from *flexus*, past participle of infinitive *flectere*, meaning "to bend, turn, turn aside."

sinuous; having curves or turns.

"The Russian ballerina's lithe body moved with a **flexuous** grace rarely found in someone her age."

Related words: **flexuously** (FLEK-shoo-əs-lee) *adverb*; **flexural** (FLEK-shər-əl) *adjective*; **flexuousness** (FLEK-shoo-əs-nis) and **flexure** (FLEK-shər) *both nouns.*

flinty (FLIN-tee)

From English **flint**, meaning "a form of silica."

1. containing flint.

"By the time we established that our collection of what we thought were valuable stones was almost exclusively **flinty** rock, it was time to give up and get back to the city."

2. obdurate; stern; unyielding; hardhearted.

"Our newest warden had a **flinty** manner that was exactly what we were looking for in a person who would have to spend most of his time refusing earnest requests from staff and prisoners."

Related words: **flintily** (FLIN-ti-lee) *adverb*; **flintiness** (FLIN-tee-nis) *noun.*

fluvial (FLOO-vee-əl)

From Latin *fluvialis*, from *fluvius* "river," + *-alis*, an adjectival suffix.

Also given as **fluviatile** (FLOO-vee-ə-til).

pertaining to a river; found in a river.

"We spent the afternoon on the riverbank taking pictures of the **fluvial** plants we saw growing there."

footloose (FUUT-loos)
From American **foot** + **loose.**

unencumbered; free to move about.

"Once Emily's husband died, she felt **footloose** and from then on did exactly what she pleased, always telling herself she was completely happy and not realizing how lonely she felt."

foppish (FOP-ish)
From English **fop,** meaning "a dandy," + **-ish,** an adjectival suffix meaning "somewhat."

excessively fastidious, particularly in behavior and dress.

"Once James was promoted to manager, he suddenly became ridiculously **foppish** and was mocked behind his back."

Related words: **foppishly** (FOP-ish-lee) *adverb*; **fop** (fop), **foppery** (FOP-ə-ree), and **foppishness** (FOP-ish-nis) *all nouns.*

forensic (fə-REN-sik)
From Latin *forensis,* meaning "public, of the marketplace."

1. argumentative, rhetorical; suited to argumentation; connected with the law or public debate.

"It was while Jonathan was quite young that we began to be subjected to his affinity for endless argumentation and soon became aware of his remarkable **forensic** skills."

2. dealing with the application of scientific knowledge to problems of law.

"With the growing acceptance of DNA as legal evidence, **forensic** biology has reached new heights of public awareness."

Related words: **forensically** (fə-REN-si-kə-lee) *adverb*; **forensicality** (fə-REN-si-KAL-i-tee) and **forensics** (fə-REN-siks) *both nouns.*

formic (FOR-mik)
From Latin *formica,* meaning "an ant."

of or pertaining to ants.

"Every spring there is a **formic** onslaught on our peonies, but the flowers appear unharmed by it."

Related words: **formicary** (FOR-mi-KER-ee), **formicarium** (FOR-mi-KAIR-ee-əm), and **formication** (FOR-mi-KAY-shən) *all nouns.*

fortuitous (for-TOO-i-təs)

From Latin *fortuitus*, meaning "accidental"; perhaps related to *fors, fortis*, meaning "chance, luck."

As you probably know, the big pitfall is thinking that **fortuitous** and **fortunate** are synonyms. They are not.

1. accidental: happening by chance.

"First in my day of **fortuitous** encounters was a meeting with my son Dick, in from London, in a bar in Seattle, where I had gone on business that morning; second, as we sat with drinks, his best friend, a New Yorker like me, came in completely unannounced and asked to sit with us."

2. INCORRECTLY: lucky, fortunate.

"How **fortuitous** it was that we met that day!"

Sentence 2 illustrates a well-known and incorrect use of **fortuitous,** a word easy to read incorrectly as **fortunate.** In the opinion of the writer, this was the unhappy result of a person's reading of a word he did not immediately understand and firmly resisted looking up in a dictionary.

After uncounted repetitions of this incorrect definition—with the kind compliance of so-called *descriptive* lexicographers who insist they are not de facto arbiters of usage but really are—this incorrect definition eventually made its way into one of the leading American dictionaries. Once there, of course, it soon was stolen by other lexicographers for their own submissive—they call it *descriptive*—dictionaries. Alas.

Why are these dictionaries here called submissive? Because their writers quietly accept any outrage and, when the outrage has been repeated sufficiently, submit to it openly and slip it into their dictionaries. They are the Little Jack Horners of dictionary writing. Faced with a chance to interpret a word in a novel sense, they stick in a thumb, pull out a linguistic plum, and say, "What a good boy am I!"

The result is that anyone who writes of how **fortuitous** something may be, is telling us how accidental it was. Now really! How accidental can anything be?

A happening or minor event can be accidental, but not more or less accidental—even though the illiterates among us are apt to characterize an event as "completely accidental" and the like. More properly, then, encounters, discoveries, and the like can be **fortunate,** even more or less **fortunate,** but not more or less accidental.

Related words: **fortuitously** (for-TOO-i-təs-lee) *adverb;* **fortuity** (for-TOO-i-tee) and **fortuitousness** (for-TOO-i-təs-nis) *both nouns.*

fortunate. *See* **fortuitous.**

frabjous (FRAB-jəs)

From a coinage, perhaps suggesting **fabulous and delicious,** in *Through the Looking-Glass,* by C. L. Dodgson, a nineteenth-century mathematician writing under the pseudonym Lewis Carroll.

first-class; wonderful, elegant.

"Carroll's immortal words were 'O **frabjous** day! Callooh! Callay!' so what could be as good?"

Related word: **frabjously** (FRAB-jəs-lee) *adverb.*

fractious (FRAK-shəs)

From English **fraction,** meaning "a rupture or interruption (obsolete meanings)" + **-ous,** an adjectival suffix.

1. of a child: unruly; stubborn.

   "In my childhood I was known for my **fractious** ways, never missing a chance to be contrary and otherwise difficult."

2. of an adult: petulant; irritable; quick to anger.

   "Adulthood and its responsibilities have not improved him a bit; he is the same **fractious** fellow he always was."

Related words: **fractiously** (FRAK-shəs-lee) *adverb;* **fractiousness** (FRAK-shəs-nis) *noun.*

frangible (FRAN-jə-bəl)

From Middle English, from Latin infinitive *frangere,* meaning "to shatter, break."

breakable; capable of being broken; easily broken.

"Almost everything in the china shop is **frangible,** and signs here and there warn customers, 'If you break it, you've bought it.'"

Related words: **frangibility** (FRAN-jə-BIL-i-tee) *adverb;* **frangibleness** (FRAN-jə-bəl-nis) *noun.*

frenetic (fri-NET-ik)

From Middle English *frenetik,* meaning "insane," from Latin *phreneticus,* meaning "delirious"; from Greek *phrenetikós.*

Also given as **frenetical** and **phrenetical** (both pronounced fri-NET-i-kəl).

frenzied; frantic.

"Once the great ship began to sink, delirium set in and **frenetic** activity overwhelmed the crew, which until then, had been commendably calm and composed."

Related words: **frenetically** (fri-NET-i-kə-lee) *adverb*; **freneticism** (fri-NET-i-sizm) *noun*.

friable (FRĪ-ə-bəl)

From Latin *friabilis*, meaning "crumbly," from infinitive *friare*, meaning "to crumble into small pieces."

easily crumbled or pulverized.

"Alfred trenched his many acres, laid pipe in the trenches, and then covered them, thus draining the land and making it suitably **friable** for all his young apple trees."

Related words: **friability** (FRĪ-ə-BIL-ə-tee) and **friableness** (FRĪ-ə-bəl-nis) *both nouns*.

fribble (FRIB-əl)

Origin unknown.

frivolous; trifling, foolish, ridiculous.

"Newspaper commentators are accusing one of the candidates of giving the voters **fribble** campaigning, for example, running commercials showing how much he likes children."

Related words: **fribble** (FRIB-əl) *verb*; **fribbler** (FRIB-lər) *noun*.

frigorific (FRIG-ə-RIF-ik)

From Latin *frigorificus*, meaning "cooling"; from *frigus*, meaning "cold; death; indifference."

cooling: causing or producing cold.

"The **frigorific** influence of Arctic ice on the temperature of the rest of the globe, particularly that of the world's oceans, is beginning to be understood."

fructiferous (fruk-TIF-ər-əs)

From Latin *fructiferus*, meaning "fruit-bearing," from Latin *fructus*, meaning "fruit."

bearing or producing fruit.

"Some tropical regions are known for their **fructiferous** trees, which are said to produce bountiful crops almost from their first year."

Related words: **fructiferously** (fruk-TIF-ər-əs-lee) *adverb*; **fructification** (FRUK-tə-fi-KAY-shən) *noun*; **fructificative** (FRUK-tə-fi-KAY-tiv) and **fructuous** (FRUK-choo-əs) *both adjectives*; **fructify** (FRUK-tə-FY) *verb*.

frugivorous (froo-JIV-ər-əs)
From Latin *frux*, meaning "fruit," + *-vorus*, a combining form meaning "devouring."

eating or feeding on fruit.

"**Frugivorous** mammals, which eat nothing but fruit, are said unreliably to produce meat of excellent taste and quality for humans."

Related word: **frugivore** (FROO-jə-VOR) *noun*.

fulgent (FUL-jənt)
From Latin *fulgens*, present participle of infinitive *fulgere*, meaning "to flash, shine; be illustrious."

resplendent; dazzling, shining brightly.

"In their **fulgent** gowns, perfect for the spotlights on the ceiling high above them, the debutantes took the ball by storm as they danced with their dates."

Related words: **fulgently** (FUL-jənt-lee) *adverb*; **fulgentness** (FUL-jənt-nis) *noun*.

Usually given as **refulgent,** which see.

fulgurous (FUL-gyər-əs)
From Latin *fulgur*, meaning "lightning; splendor."

resembling lightning; charged with lightning.

"During dinner we were fortunate to observe an awesomely **fulgurous** display in the western sky."

Related words: **fulgurant** (FUL-gyər-ənt), **fulgurating** (FUL-gyə-RAY-ting) *both adjectives*.

fuliginous (fyoo-LIJ-ə-nəs)
From Latin *fuliginosus*, meaning "full of soot"; from *fuligo*, meaning "soot," + *-osus*, an adjectival suffix meaning "full of."

sooty; smoky; blackened with soot.

"Manchester, England, long had been notorious for its yellow, **fuliginous** air and coughing residents."

Related words: **fuliginously** (fyoo-LIJ-ə-nəs-lee) *adverb*; **fuliginousness** (fyoo-LIJ-ə-nəs-nis) *noun*.

fulminant (FUL-mə-nənt)

From Latin *fulminans*, present participle of infinitive *fulminare*, meaning "to lighten, strike with lightning."

fulminating; highly explosive; suddenly occurring.

"Cynical epidemiologists claim that the **fulminant** West Nile virus, which thus far has hardly ever killed anybody, owes much of its virulence and notoriety to the exotic name it sports."

Related words: **fulminate** (FUL-mə-NAYT) *verb*; **fulminator** (FUL-mə-NAY-tər) and **fulmination** (FUL-mə-NAY-shən) *both nouns*; **fulminatory** (FUL-mə-NAY-tə-ree) and **fulminic** (ful-MIN-ik) *both adjectives*.

fulsome (FUUL-səm)

Possibly from Middle English *fulsom*, meaning "copious, cloying." A word of various modern and obsolete meanings.

Today's meanings demonstrate adequately the generally negative tone of the word. Yet, many modern readers and writers—with the complicity of many of their dastardly dictionaries—misinterpret **fulsome** as an approving term, roughly defining it as "copious." Too bad.

1. of a person: generally offensive, particularly in regard to aesthetics or morals.

"When he finally made his political feelings clear, we all could see he was a **fulsome** liar."

2. of a thing: offensive to good taste.

"After waiting many weeks for an invitation to view the newly decorated apartment, we were finally rewarded with a display of the **fulsome** vulgarity for which their designer was famous."

Related words: **fulsomely** (FUUL-səm-lee) *adverb*; **fulsomeness** (FUUL-səm-nis) *noun*.

fungible (FUN-jə-bəl)

From Medieval Latin *fungibilis*, from Latin infinitive *fungi*, meaning "to perform or discharge; do."

of goods, etc.: freely exchangeable for something else; interchangeable.

"The ultimate example of a **fungible** item is money, especially the money of a firmly established country of excellent credit."

Related word: **fungibility** (FUN-jə-BIL-ə-tee) *noun*.

fuscous (FUS-kəs)

From Latin *fuscus*, meaning "dark, dusky."

of a dark or somber hue; brownish gray.

"He took no notice of his wife's depressed state until he realized she had abandoned the colorful prints she formerly enjoyed and was wearing nothing but **fuscous** clothes."

fusty (FUS-tee)

From Middle English and Old French *fusti*, meaning "wine cask, tree trunk"; from Latin *fustis*, meaning "stick, club, cudgel."

1. of food: moldy.

"I wouldn't mind a **fusty** cold lamb if the chef at least tried to disguise it with a hot, spicy sauce."

2. of places: stuffy, close.

"When we finally got rooms at the inn, they were so **fusty** we had to open the windows wide to air them out."

3. of persons or styles: old-fashioned, old fogyish.

"If you insist on wearing those **fusty** tweed jackets everywhere, you had better become accustomed to knowing no one will ever hire you to design anything at all modern."

Related words: **fustily** (FUS-ti-lee) *adverb*; **fustiness** (FUS-ti-nis) *noun*.

G

gainful (GAYN-fəl)

From English **gain,** a well-known word, + **-ful,** an adjectival suffix meaning "characterized by." A happier word than **gainless** (GAYN-lis), its antonym.

In most cases in which **gainful** is used, it characterizes activities generally assumed to be examples of lucrative gain, apparently leaving other types of gains for the moralist.

profitable; lucrative; remunerative.

"She took the volunteer job that was offered in hope that in no more than a few months it would lead to **gainful** employment."

Related words: **gainfully** (GAYN-fə-lee) *adverb;* **gainfulness** (GAYN-fəl-nis) *noun.*

gainly (GAYN-lee)

Possibly a back formation from **ungainly,** meaning "clumsy; homely."

of appearance or behavior: graceful; handsome; comely.

"All she could remember of her younger brother was that he had been **gainly** and, unlike many others his age, always obliging."

Related word: **gainliness** (GAYN-lee-nis) *noun.*

galactopoietic (gə-LAK-tə-poy-ET-ik)

From English **galacto-,** a combining form meaning "milk," + **-poietic,** a combining form meaning "making."

increasing the production of milk.

"She was given what they said would be a **galactopoietic** diet, suggesting it would help her nurse the baby successfully."

Related word: **galactopoiesis** (gə-LAK-tə-poy-EE-sis) *noun.*

gamesome (GAYM-səm)

From English **game,** meaning "pastime," + **-some,** an adjectival suffix, together meaning "like a game."

playful; sportive; full of play.

"Evelyn, as **gamesome** as ever, claimed she surely would beat the boys at any sport they chose."

Related words: **gamesomely** (GAYM-səm-lee) *adverb*; **gamesomeness** (GAYM-səm-nis) *noun*.

garrulous (GAR-ə-ləs)

From Latin *garrulus,* meaning "talkative, babbling"; from infinitive *garrire,* meaning "to chatter."

1. of a person: excessively talkative, especially about trivial matters.

"The chairperson of the committee had to dismiss the **garrulous** aide because her chatter interfered with their work."

2. of a speech or paper: diffuse; excessively wordy.

"Al was furious when he saw the bill submitted by the speechwriter for the boring and **garrulous** speech he had written."

Related words: **garrulity** (gə-ROO-li-tee) and **garrulousness** (GAR-ə-ləs-nis) *both nouns*; **garrulously** (GAR-ə-ləs-lee) *adverb*.

gelid (JEL-id)

From Latin *gelidus,* meaning "icy cold; numb."

1. of temperature: extremely cold.

"All he knew for certain was that the dessert had to be **gelid** in order for it to set properly."

2. of people and their emotions: cold as ice.

"We knew Joe had discovered our prank when we saw his **gelid** expression."

Related words: **gelidly** (JEL-id-lee) *adverb*; **gelidity** (jə-LID-i-tee) and **gelidness** (JEL-id-nis) *both nouns*.

geminate (JEM-ə-nit)

From Latin *geminatus,* meaning "doubled," past participle of *geminare,* meaning "to repeat, double"; from *geminus,* "a twin."

Also given as **geminated** (JEM-ə-NAYT-id).

duplicated; twin; combined in pairs.

"After long consideration of all the photographs they had, the astronomers agreed that what they were seeing was the latest in a series of new **geminate** stars."

Related words: **geminate** (JEM-ə-NAYT) *verb*; **geminately** (JEM-ə-nit-lee) *adverb*; **gemination** (JEM-ə-NAY-shən) *noun*.

generic (jə-NER-ik)
From Latin *genus*, meaning "kind, sort, species."

1. general; applicable to all members of a specific class, etc.

"His art history teacher asked the class to compile a documented list of **generic** traits found in the work of outstanding eighteenth-century Flemish painters."

2. unprotected by trademark.

"I asked my physician whether I could buy a low-priced **generic** drug instead of the expensive proprietary drug he recommended."

Related words: **generically** (jə-NER-i-kə-lee) *adverb*; **genericness** (jə-NER-ik-nis) *noun*.

german (JUR-mən)
From Middle English *germain* from Latin *germanus*, meaning "of the same parents"; from Latin *germen*, meaning "bud or branch; embryo."

1. closely related; of the same parent.

"Few people know that David and I, because we appear to be unrelated, are actually brothers-**german.**"

2. first cousin; of a son or daughter of one's uncle or aunt.

"Uncle Max and Aunt Mary were so prolific that I can boast of having eleven cousins-**german.**"

germane (jər-MAYN)
From Middle English *germain*, meaning "having the same parents"; from Latin *germanus* (see etymology of **german** above).

of a statement, etc.: fitting; at the same time both relevant and pertinent.

"Nothing he ever said was uninteresting, but the fact is that things he said often were not **germane,** and much as we would have liked to understand his discussion, we really could not."

Related word: **germanely** (jər-MAYN-lee) *adverb*; **germaneness** (jər-MAYN-nis) *noun*.

gestic (JES-tik)

From Latin *gestus*, meaning "gesticulation, gesture; movement of the limbs"; from *gesta*, meaning "exploits."

Also given as **gestical** (JES-ti-kəl).

of or pertaining to bodily movement, especially in dancing.

"Her **gestic** magic entranced her Lincoln Center devotees, astonishing them with the grace and ease she showed in all her movements."

Related words: **gest** and **geste** (both pronounced "jest") *nouns*.

glabrous (GLAY-brəs)

From Latin *glaber*, meaning "smooth, bald."

Also given as **glabrate** (GLAY-brayt).

in science: hairless; smooth-surfaced.

"She began to specialize in completely **glabrous** houseplants after she found they were often overlooked in most private collections."

Related word: **glabrescent** (glay-BRES-ənt) *adjective*.

glaucous (GLAW-kəs)

From Latin *glaucus*, meaning "bluish gray; silvery"; from Greek *glaukós*.

greenish blue; bluish gray.

"In late August, the field's purple grapes were suddenly covered with a **glaucous** powder, signaling to all believers that the field could be harvested in three or four weeks."

Related word: **glaucously** (GLAW-kəs-lee) *adverb*.

glutinous (GLOOT-n-əs)

From Latin *glutinosus*, meaning "sticky, gluey."

Not to be confused with the well-understood **gluttonous** (GLUT-n-əs), "compulsive overeaters," from Latin infinitive *glutire*, "to wolf down, swallow."

sticky; viscid; gluey.

"Unfortunately, the child put his hands on the fresh paint and found that its somewhat **glutinous** surface yielded enough pleasure to invite repeated attempts to leave his mark."

Related words: **glutinously** (GLOOT-n-əs-lee) *adverb;* **glutinous-ness** (GLOOT-n-əs-nis) *noun.*

gluttonous. *See* **glutinous.**

glyptic (GLIP-tik)
From Greek *glyptikós,* meaning "of engraving"; from infinitive *glyphein,* meaning "to engrave."

of gems: pertaining to engraving or carving.

"As the number of highly publicized jewel thefts increased, there arose a demand for persons skilled in creating tiny **glyptic** identifications that would thwart thieves."

Related words: **glyph** (glif), **glyptics** (GLIP-tiks), **glyptograph** (GLIP-tə-GRAF), **glyptography** (glip-TOG-rə-fee), and **glyptographer** (glip-TOG-rə-fər) *all nouns.*

gnathonic (na-THON-ik)
From Latin *gnathonicus,* meaning "subservient"; from the name *Gnatho,* a fawning character in a Roman comedy by Terence, second century B.C.

sycophantic; bootlicking; parasitical.

"The outgoing vice president fortunately had reached the stage at which he no longer saw it necessary to act the **gnathonic** jester, seemingly agreeing with everything the boss said even before he said it."

Related word: **gnathonically** (na-THON-i-kal-ee) *adverb.*

goutish (GOW-tish, rhymes with *loutish*)
From Middle English *goute,* from Latin *gutta,* meaning "a drop, a speck," + *-ish,* an adjectival suffix meaning "belonging to."

affected with or suffering from gout; swollen as if from gout.

"The patient may exhibit an excess of uric acid in the blood, giving rise to an excruciating **goutish** pain in the big toe of a foot that once encountered is never forgotten."

Related words: **gout** (gowt) and **goutiness** (GOW-tee-nis) *both nouns;* **gouty** (GOW-tee) *adjective;* **goutily** (GOW-ti-lee) *adverb.*

gramineous (grə-MIN-ee-əs)
From Latin *gramineus,* meaning "grassy." *See also* **graminivorous.**

grassy.

"After we finished building our house, we established a **gramineous** field around it and fenced it in to accommodate our dogs and horses."

Related word: **gramineousness** (grə-MIN-ee-əs-nis) *noun.*

graminivorous (GRAM-ə-NIV-ər-əs)

From Latin *gramen*, meaning "grass," + *-i-* + English **-vorous,** a combining form meaning "eating."

feeding on grass.

"Range-fed steers are **graminivorous** animals, yielding tasteful if not always tender beef."

grandiloquent (gran-DIL-ə-kwənt)

From English **grandiloquence**, meaning "lofty speech"; from Latin *grandiloquus*, meaning "grand speaker, boaster."

of a person: characterized by swollen or pompous speech.

"At the convention all those who spoke, whether future local postmasters or illiterate state governors, were **grandiloquent** lackeys coached by the speechwriters of the party nominee."

Related words: **grandiloquence** (gran-DIL-ə-kwəns) *noun*; **grandiloquently** (gran-DIL-ə-kwənt-lee) *adverb.*

gratuitous (grə-TOO-i-təs)

From Latin *gratuitus*, meaning "free, gratuitous."

free; given without payment or other remuneration or justification.

"Seemingly without justification he always impugned the motives of other guests with his **gratuitous** insults."

Related words: **gratuitously** (grə-TOO-i-təs-lee) *adverb*; **gratuitousness** (grə-TOO-i-təs-nis) and **gratuity** (grə-TOO-i-tee) *both nouns.*

gravid (GRAV-id)

From Latin *gravidus*, meaning "pregnant, full."

pregnant.

"All the guppies in my tank of tropical fish appeared to be **gravid** during the latter part of my wife's first pregnancy."

Related words: **gravidity** (grə-VID-i-tee) and **gravidness** (GRAV-id-nis) *both nouns*; **gravidly** (GRAV-id-lee) *adverb.*

gregarious (gri-GAR-ee-əs)

From Latin *gregarius*, meaning "common; belonging to a flock."

1. of persons: fond of company; sociable.

   "No matter where they are, my **gregarious** brothers always strike up conversations with strangers."

2. of animals: living in flocks or herds of others of the same species.

   "He particularly liked a village in Wales where serene, **gregarious** sheep could be observed wherever one decided to live."

   Related words: **gregariously** (gri-GAR-ee-əs-lee) *adverb*; **gregariousness** (gri-GAR-ee-əs-nis) *noun*.

grueling (GROO-ə-ling)
From the past participle of an obsolete English verb **gruel,** meaning "to exhaust or disable."

punishing to the point of exhaustion; exhausting.

"The **grueling** race was over, but the exhausted athletes were unable to speak, much less hold press conferences."

Related word: **gruelingly** (GROO-ə-ling-lee) *adverb*.

guileless (GĪL-lis)
From English **guile,** meaning "insidious cunning," + **-less,** an adjectival suffix meaning "without."

straightforward; frank; innocent; devoid of guile.

"Jonny soon learned not to be so **guileless** with his older siblings after he had confessed to them that he deliberately manipulated them."

Related words: **guile** (gīl) *noun*; **guileful** (GĪL-fəl) *adjective*; **guilefulness** (GĪL-fəl-nis) *noun*; **guilelessly** (GĪL-lis-lee) *adverb*; **guilelessness** (GĪL-lis-nis) *noun*.

guttiform (GUT-ə-form)
From Latin *gutta*, meaning "a drop," + *-form*, together meaning "shaped like a drop."

drop shaped.

"The slow drip froze and thawed alternately, leading to **guttiform** shapes that gradually covered the entire surface."

H

hackneyed (HAK-need)

From a place-name in the county of Middlesex, England. In Middle English called *hakeney* and in English called **Hackney.**

The adjective **hackney** meant "let out," and the verb **hackney** meant "make stale, usually by overuse." **Hackneyed** is the past participle of the verb **hackney.**

banal; made trite, stale, commonplace.

"My sister and I groaned quietly behind our uncle's back at the boring, **hackneyed** jokes with which he regaled us."

hagridden (HAG-RID-n)

Perhaps from Middle English *hagge*, meaning "witch,"+ *ridden*, a combining form meaning "overwhelmed by," past participle of "to ride."

harassed by a nightmare.

"My **hagridden** nights, populated with shrieking witches, are leaving me tormented and unrefreshed, scarcely able to face the demands of a new day."

Related words: **hagride** (HAG-RĪD) *verb*; **hagrider** (HAG-rīd-ər) *noun*.

halcyon (HAL-see-ən)

From Latin *halcyon*, from Greek *halkyón*, meaning "kingfisher"; from *hals*, "the sea," + *kuo*, "to brood on."

Ancients believed the kingfisher laid its eggs on the surface of the sea and incubated them for two weeks, called "the halcyon days," during which, according to tradition, the waves were always unruffled; hence the expression **halcyon days** to describe a serene time.

tranquil, peaceful; undisturbed; prosperous.

"The sudden cessation of warfare combined with the unexpected beginnings of a vigorous economy had given us **halcyon** days."

hapless (HAP-lis)

From Old Norse *happ*, meaning "luck or chance; good luck."

Another of those terms for which one would expect to have an antonym. Yet no one is ever known as *hapful*, which would be a good name for a Las Vegas gambling house—or gaming casino, as it surely would prefer to be called.

unlucky, unfortunate; luckless.

"The casino was full of gamblers, most of them **hapless** veterans, the rest a scant sprinkling of lucky ones."

Related words: **haplessly** (HAP-lis-lee) *adverb*; **haplessness** (HAP-lis-nis) *noun*.

hardscrabble (HAHRD-SKRAB-əl)

From American **hard,** meaning "difficult,"+ the verb **scrabble,** meaning "to scratch out."

demanding; yielding little in return for hard work.

"Jess eked out enough income from the **hardscrabble** farm he and his father worked for many years to enable him to go to college."

haughty (HAW-tee)

From Middle English *haute*, from Medieval French *haut*, both from Latin *altus*, meaning "high."

high in one's own estimation; proud, arrogant; snobbish.

"How strange it was that someone born as well as Patricia and educated at the finest schools could be made to feel inferior by a **haughty** receptionist."

Related words: **haughtily** (HAW-ti-lee) *adverb*; **haughtiness** (HAW-tee-nis) *noun*.

hedonic (hee-DON-ik)

From Greek *hedonikós*, meaning "pleasurable."

pertaining to pleasure or pleasantness.

"When he began to recover from his cardiac operation, he looked on his new life as a **hedonic** experience."

Related words: **hedonics** (hee-DON-iks) and **hedonism** (HEED-n-ɪz-əm) *both nouns*; **hedonically** (hee-DON-ik-əl-ee) *adverb.*

heinous (HAY-nəs)

From Middle English *heynous*, from French *haineux*, meaning "hateful."

of persons or their acts: odious; abominable.

"The close of the twentieth century, unmatched for cruelty, has brought no cessation of **heinous** crimes against humanity."

Related words: **heinously** (HAY-nəs-lee) *adverb*; **heinousness** (HAY-nəs-nis) *noun.*

hemathermal (HE-mə-THUR-məl)

From English **hema-,** a combining form meaning "blood," + **thermal,** meaning "pertaining to heat."

Also given as **homoiothermal** (hoh-MOY-ə-THUR-məl).

warm-blooded; characterized by having a relatively constant temperature.

"Humans, along with other mammals, are **hemathermal** creatures, making them able to thrive in an enormous range of ambient temperatures."

Hemingwayesque (HEM-ing-way-ESK)

From the name of **Ernest Hemingway,** twentieth-century American novelist and short-story writer, + **-esque,** an adjectival suffix indicating resemblance.

characteristic of the style or works of Hemingway, direct and unadorned.

"In what he mistakenly hoped would become a **Hemingwayesque** story, spare and replete with simple, declarative sentences, the young writer revealed his total lack of talent and individuality."

herbivorous (hur-BIV-ər-əs)

From Modern Latin *herbivorus*, meaning "herb-eating."

plant-eating.

"Cows, large **herbivorous** animals that appear in summer to eat nothing but grass, must spend many hours every day munching away on their feed."

Related words: **herbivore** (HUR-bə-VOR) *noun*; **herbivorously** (hur-BIV-ər-əs-lee) *adverb.*

hermaphroditic (hur-MAF-rə-DIT-ik)

From Latin *hermaphroditus* from Greek *hermaphróditos,* both of which mean "hermaphrodite," also, capitalized, the proper name of the son of Hermes and Aphrodite.

And what is a **hermaphrodite**? A person or other creature that contains sexual characteristics of both male and female. The adjective is also given as **hermaphroditical** (hur-MAF-rə-DIT-i-kəl).

combining male and female characteristics.

"Our cousins, in their first trip to the big city, said they wanted to see a show featuring **hermaphroditic** performers."

Related words: **hermaphrodite** (hur-MAF-rə-DĪT) and **hermaphroditism** (hur-MAF-rə-dī-TIZ-əm) *both nouns.*

hermeneutic (HUR-mə-NOO-tik)

From Greek *hermeneútikós,* meaning "skilled in interpreting"; from *hermeneús,* "an interpreter"; from *Hermes,* messenger of the gods.

Also given as **hermeneutical** (HUR-mə-NOO-ti-kəl).

concerned with interpretation; explanatory; interpretive.

"The **hermeneutic** skill he showed in his celebrated lecture on interpreting poetry dazzled the entire faculty."

Related words: **hermeneutically** (HUR-mə-NOO-ti-kə-lee) *adverb;* **hermeneutics** (HUR-mə-NOO-tiks) *noun.*

hermitic (hur-MIT-ik). *See* **troglodytic.**

heterochthonous (HET-ə-ROK-thə-nəs)

From Greek *hetero-,* a combining form meaning "different," from Greek *héteros,* meaning "the other," + *chthón,* meaning "earth," + *-ous,* an adjectival suffix.

Much less common than the adjective **autochthonous** (aw-TOK-thə-nəs), which means "native, indigenous."

foreign; not indigenous, not native.

"Once the ancient city had been uncovered, we traced its successive invasions by foreign forces through examining fossilized remains of **heterochthonous** plants, giving us a botanical map of the movement of ancient armies making their way along the Mediterranean."

heterodox (HET-ər-ə-DOKS)

From Greek *heteródoxos,* meaning "of another opinion"; from Greek *hetero-*, a combining form meaning "different," + *dóx*, meaning "an opinion," + *-os*, an adjectival suffix.

of persons, of beliefs: unorthodox; holding unorthodox ideas.

"In the first speech the new principal gave before our parent's club he pleased some parents with his **heterodox** ideas and filled others with apprehension."

Related words: **heterodoxy** (HET-ər-ə-DOK-see) *noun*; **heterodoxly** (HET-ər-ə-DOKS-lee) *adverb*.

heuristic (hyuu-RIS-tik)

From New Latin *heuristicus*, from Greek *heuriskein*, meaning "to find out"; the Latin *-isticus* is an adjectival suffix meaning "in other words."

serving to find out or discover (something).

"Obviously, the **heuristic** problems selected by the instructor were welcome, because students had not learned anything from the rote exercises they had previously been doing."

Related word: **heuristically** (hyuu-RIS-ti-klee) *adverb*.

hibernal (hī-BUR-nl)

From Latin *hibernalis*, from *hibernus*, meaning "wintry," + *-alis*, an adjectival suffix appearing mostly in scientific terms.

wintry; pertaining to winter; appearing in winter.

"Some of the animals began appearing in their **hibernal** coats, and some then retired into their winter caves, a clear sign that the rest of us had better leave for home."

Related words: **hibernate** (HĪ-bər-NAYT) *verb*; **hibernation** (HĪ-bər-NAY-shən) and **hibernator** (HĪ-bər-NAY-tər) *both nouns*.

hircine (HUR-sīn)

From the Latin adjective *hircinus*, meaning "of a goat."

1. resembling a goat in color, smell, etc.

"The goat cheese farm Miles established gave off a distinctly **hircine** aroma that made it possible for a visitor to identify the spread without having to find a direction sign."

2. lustful.

"Harry was surprised to find that his adolescent companions referred to him as **Hircine** Harry, suggesting he yearned for girls."

hirsute (hur-SOOT)

From Latin *hirsutus*, meaning "shaggy; bristly; uncouth."

1. hairy; having rough or shaggy hair.

"In the days when it was cool to go about **hirsute,** I sometimes had trouble recognizing my own sons."

2. pertaining to hair.

"Most men who are serious about their desire to find suitable employment take pains to appear clean-shaven, totally devoid of **hirsute** ornament."

Related words: **hirsuteness** (hur-SOOT-nis) and **hirsutism** (hur-SOO-tiz-əm) *both nouns.*

histrionic (HIS-tree-ON-ik)

From Late Latin *histrionicus*, meaning "of actors," from *histrio*, "an actor," or from *histrionalis*, "of an actor."

Also given in English as **histrionical** (HIS-tree-ON-i-kəl).

1. overly dramatic; hypocritical; deceitful.

"John's **histrionic** final speech to the jury is said to have lost his case."

2. dramatic; theatrical.

"The young mother proved no match for the lachrymose demands of her **histrionic** daughter, who was able to turn her tears on and off at will."

Related words: **histrionically** (HIS-tree-ON-i-kə-lee) *adverb;* **histrionics** (HIS-tree-ON-iks) *noun.*

homoiothermal. *See* **hemathermal.**

hortatory (HOR-tə-TOR-ee)

From Late Latin *hortatorius*, meaning "encouraging," from Latin infinitive *hortari*, "to encourage."

Also given as **hortative** (HOR-tə-tiv).

characterized by exhorting, encouraging; pertaining to exhortation, encouragement.

"I found reasoning and dialogue more effective than **hortatory** speeches."

Related words: **hortatorily** (HOR-tə-TOR-i-lee) and **hortatively** (HOR-tə-tiv-lee) *both adverbs.*

huffish (HUF-ish)

From English **huff,** meaning "a fit of resentment or petulance," + **-ish,** an adjectival suffix meaning "like."

arrogant; insolent; bullying; petulant.

"His father would turn **huffish** at some fancied insult—for example, an imagined challenge to his intelligence—and make the rest of family dinners impossible to enjoy."

Related words: **huffy** (HUF-ee) *adjective*; **huffishly** (HUF-ish-lee) and **huffily** (HUF-i-lee) *both adverbs*; **huffishness** (HUF-ish-nis) and **huffiness** (HUF-i-nis) *both nouns.*

I

iatric (ī-A-trik)

> From Greek *iatrikós*, meaning "of healing," from *iatrós*, "healer, physician."

> Also given in English as **iatrical** (ī-AT-ri-kəl).

> medical, medicinal; pertaining to a physician or medicine.

>> "The **iatric** art has helped mankind by reducing pain, preventing illness, and curing undesirable conditions."

See **iatrogenic.**

iatrogenic (ī-A-trə-JEN-ik)

> From English **iatro-**, a combining form meaning "healer, physician, medicine," + *-genic*, a combining form meaning "causing."

> of a medical condition: unintentionally caused by the diagnosis or treatment of a physician.

>> "Some of our major hospitals have seen fit to establish departments that monitor physicians' medical practices and evaluate patients' complaints of what are considered to be **iatrogenic** conditions."

> Related word: **iatrogenicity** (Ī-A-trə-jə-NIS-i-tee) *noun.*

See also **iatric.**

idoneous (ī-DOH-nee-əs)

> From Latin *idoneus*, meaning "fit, proper, suitable."

> apt; fit; suitable.

>> "On the basis of their **idoneous** qualifications, all three finalists were given four-month appointments as summer interns to determine how they would respond to the demands of a working environment."

Related words: **idoneity** (ID-n-EE-i-tee) and **idoneousness** (ī-DOH-nee-əs-nis) *both nouns.*

idyllic (ī-DIL-ik)

From English *idyll,* from Latin *idyllium,* from Greek *eidyllion,* all meaning "a short descriptive poem."

charmingly simple or rustic; forming a suitable theme for a poem.

"For two blissful weeks we led an **idyllic** existence in the Vermont countryside."

Related words: **idyll** (ĪD-l) and **idyllist** (ĪD-l-ist) *both nouns;* **idyllically** (ī-DIL-i-klee) *adverb.*

ignescent (ig-NES-ənt)

From Latin *ignescens,* present participle of *ignescere,* meaning "to burst into flames; burn."

bursting into flames; emitting real or figurative sparks.

"He was blessed with the type of **ignescent** personality that quickly burst into a five-alarm fire at the slightest provocation."

Related word: **igneous** (IG-nee-əs) *adjective.*

ignominious (IG-nə-MIN-ee-əs)

From Latin *ignominiosus,* meaning "degraded, disgraced; shameful."

humiliating; contemptible.

"The team's bumbling errors finally were capped by an **ignominious** kick into our own goal."

Related words: **ignominiously** (ig-nə-MIN-ee-əs-lee) *adverb;* **ignominy** (IG-nə-MIN-ee) and **ignominiousness** (ig-nə-MIN-ee-əs-nis) *both nouns.*

illicit (i-LIS-it)

From Latin *illicitus,* meaning "unlawful."

not authorized or allowed; unlawful, forbidden.

"**Illicit** production of whiskey has been known to cause deaths in my home state."

Related words: **illicitly** (i-LIS-it-lee) *adverb;* **illicitness** (i-LIS-it-nis) *noun.*

imitable (IM-i-tə-bəl)

From Latin *imitabilis,* meaning "imitable," from infinitive *imitare,* meaning "to imitate."

This adjective is nowhere near as well known as its opposite, **inimitable,** meaning "incapable of being imitated or copied." *See* **inimitable.**

capable of being imitated.

"Few of the new engineers do entirely original work, instead depending for their inspiration on the **imitable** work of their predecessors."

Related words: **imitability** (IM-i-tə-BIL-i-tee) and **imitableness** (IM-i-tə-bəl-nis) *both nouns.*

imminent (IM-ə-nənt)
From Latin *imminens,* present participle of infinitive *imminere,* meaning "to overhang; threaten."

impending; hanging over one's head; likely to occur at any moment.

"The feeling he had of **imminent** disaster proved untrue, of course, but it robbed him of the self-confidence he needed to meet all the demands we put on him."

Related words: **imminently** (IM-ə-nənt-lee) *adverb;* **imminence** (IM-ə-nəns) and **imminentness** (IM-ə-nənt-nis) *both nouns.*

immutable (i-MYOO-tə-bəl)
From Latin *immutabilis,* meaning "unalterable."

unchangeable; unalterable; changeless.

"As the final scenes of the trial played out, the only things **immutable** in the courtroom were the heavy wooden furniture and the expression on the judge's face."

Related words: **immutably** (i-MYOO-tə-blee) *adverb;* **immutability** (i-MYOO-tə-BIL-i-tee) and **immutableness** (i-MYOO-tə-bəl-nis) *both nouns.*

impassive (im-PAS-iv)
From English well-known **passive + im-,** meaning "not."

1. not subject to suffering.

"Of all the inmates in the camp, the ones who disturbed their captors most were those who managed somehow to appear **impassive** no matter how the guards tortured them."

2. apathetic; without emotion; insensible; calm, serene.

"We could read nothing in the **impassive** faces of the jury, even when grisly testimony was being given."

Related words: **impassively** (im-PAS-iv-lee) *adverb*; **impassivity** (IM-pa-SIV-i-tee) and **impassiveness** (im-PAS-iv-nis) *both nouns.*

impeachable. *See* **unimpeachable.**

impeccable (im-PEK-ə-bəl)

From Latin *impeccabilis*, meaning "faultless, free of sin"; from infinitive *peccare*, meaning "to make a mistake; go wrong; offend."

Giving us a picture of an earlier day, when sin could take several forms, not solely that of transgression against divine law.

1. not capable of or liable to sin.

"The general, albeit incorrect, perception of the attorney was that he was **impeccable** and would so remain until he died."

2. irreproachable; flawless, faultless.

"As strange as it sounds, while his manners were always **impeccable,** even on a social evening he never missed a chance to cheat at cards."

See also **peccable.**

Related words: **impeccably** (im-PEK-ə-blee) *adverb*; **impeccability** (im-PEK-ə-BIL-i-tee) *noun.*

impecunious (IM-pi-KYOO-nee-əs)

From Latin *im-*, meaning "not," + *pecuniosus*, meaning "moneyed, well-off."

poor; having no money.

"Strangely, the only happy branch of our family is the **impecunious** one, whose members never seem to worry about their apparent lack of cash."

Related words: **impecuniously** (IM-pi-KYOO-nee-əs-lee) *adverb*; **impecuniousness** (IM-pi-KYOO-nee-əs-nis) and **impecuniosity** (IM-pi-KYOO-nee-OS-i-tee) *both nouns.*

implacable (im-PLAK-ə-bəl)

From Latin *implacabilis*, meaning "unforgiving; not placable."

While the verb **placate** and the adjective **implacable** are often heard and well understood, **placable,** meaning "forgiving," is rarely encountered. It seems this is another of those English constructions in which the negative wins out over the positive. Or is it just another example of the stiff-upper-lip English locutions that make so much of sterling character?

irreconcilable; inexorable; incapable of being appeased.

"Once the republican leader fully understood all the machinations of the ousted royal family, he and his party became **implacable** enemies of despotism."

Related words: **implacably** (im-PLAK-ə-blee) *adverb*; **implacability** (im-PLAK-ə-BIL-i-tee) and **implacableness** (im-PLAK-ə-bəl-nis) *both nouns.*

implausible (im-PLAW-zə-bəl)

From English **im-,** meaning "not," + **plausible,** meaning "believable"; from Latin *plausibilis,* meaning "praiseworthy."

not plausible; not having the appearance of truth.

"His stories about his adventures at Princeton seemed **implausible,** but years later they were verified by classmates, who said they remembered every one of his wild escapades."

Related words: **implausibly** (im-PLAW-zə-blee) *adverb*; **implausibility** (im-PLAW-zə-BIL-ə-tee) and **implausibleness** (im-PLAW-zə-bəl-nis) *both nouns.*

importunate (im-POR-chə-nit)

From Latin *importunus,* meaning "unsuitable, troublesome."

1. pertinacious; persistent in solicitation; relentless.

"I dread tomorrow's visit by the committee, openly intended to harass me once more with their **importunate** demands."

2. annoying; troublesome.

"No matter how the couple tried to avoid their **importunate** creditors, at last they had to admit defeat."

Related words: **importune** (IM-por-TOON) *verb*; **importunately** (im-POR-chə-nit-lee) *adverb*; **importunateness** (im-POR-chə-nit-nis) *noun.*

impuissant (im-PYOO-ə-sənt)

From Latin *potens,* present participle of infinitive *posse,* meaning "to have power," + *im-,* prefix meaning "not"; more recently from French *puissant,* meaning "powerful," + *im-.*

feeble; weak, lacking power.

"Richard could scarcely be termed an **impuissant** monarch when all he lacked was a large retinue of strong and good friends and an ample store of good luck."

Related word: **impuissance** (im-PYOO-ə-səns) *noun.*

imputrescible (IM-pyoo-TRES-ə-bəl)

From Late Latin *imputrescibilis,* meaning "not prone to rotting; imputrescible"; from Latin infinitive *putrescere,* meaning "to rot."

A cousin of the common adjective **putrid,** from Latin *putridus,* meaning "rotten, decayed; withered."

not liable to putrefaction; incorruptible.

"An advantage of cooked food is that it is said to be more nearly **imputrescible** than untreated food."

inapposite (in-AP-ə-zit)

From English **apposite,** meaning "pertinent," + **in-,** meaning "not."

not to the point; not pertinent.

"Many of the arguments he presented were immediately found to be thoroughly **inapposite** and so were disqualified from consideration."

Related words: **inappositely** (in-AP-ə-zit-lee) *adverb*; **inappositeness** (in-AP-ə-zit-nis) *noun.*

inauspicious (IN-aw-SPISH-əs)

From Latin *auspicium,* meaning "favorable omen," + *in-,* meaning "not."

It is words like this one that take us back to the good old days when people saw omens — some good and some bad — in all sorts of things, and the rest of us paid attention to them.

The Latin name for such omens comes from *avis,* meaning "a bird" + the infinitive *specere,* meaning "to observe," and the name for the soothsayers was *auspices,* singular *auspex,* since these wise men and women, in Latin and English often called *augurs,* used birds and other phenomena to determine the meanings of such signs. And an augur would observe *auspices* to determine whether the gods favored or disfavored a proposed action.

ill-omened; unlucky, unfortunate; boding ill.

"Each Monday morning we would watch anxiously for any **inauspicious** sign on the face of our boss, apparently suggesting that business was bad and we would soon close permanently."

Related words: **inauspiciously** (IN-aw-SPISH-əs-lee) *adverb*; **inauspiciousness** (IN-aw-SPISH-əs-nis) *noun*.

inchoate (in-KOH-it)

From Latin *inchoatus,* more properly *incohatus,* past participle of *inchoare,* more properly *incohare,* meaning "to begin, start work on."

victim of a linguistic mishap.

And wouldn't life have been easier if a copyist's transposition of letters "h" and "o" had not occurred back in Latin and saddened students of two languages? But life hasn't been easier, and we are left with both etymologically incomprehensible *inch* words.

1. rudimentary; immature; not fully developed.

"We made the gross error of inviting the press in to hear our story even though our plans were still **inchoate**."

2. incipient; in an initial stage; just begun.

"As usual, Edith's **inchoate** ideas came tumbling out and were adopted immediately, when another week or two of rumination would have done wonders for us."

Related words: **inchoately** (in-KOH-it-lee) *adverb*; **inchoative** (in-KOH-ə-tiv) *adjective*; **inchoation** (IN-koh-AY-shən) and **inchoateness** (in-KOH-it-nis) *both nouns*.

incredulous (in-KREJ-ə-ləs)

From Latin *incredulus,* from *in-,* meaning "not," + *credulus,* meaning "believing."

Not to be confused with **incredible,** meaning "unbelievable," a word universally known and widely misapplied by broadcasters and sports enthusiasts, who contaminate almost everything they touch. They apparently think misuse of **incredulous** earns more brownie points than correct use of **incredible**.

Whatever they think, people who find it hard to believe something are correctly said to be **incredulous,** while the stories you tell that are hard to believe are properly **incredible**.

skeptical; unbelieving; not ready to believe; showing disbelief.

"Pat's **incredulous** stare at the witness then giving testimony did not go unnoticed by the jury."

Related words: **incredulously** (in-KREJ-ə-ləs-lee) *adverb*; **incredulity** (IN-kri-DOO-li-tee) and **incredulousness** (in-KEJ-ə-ləs-nis) *both nouns*.

inculpable (in-KUL-pə-bəl)

From Latin *inculpabilis,* meaning "not culpable."

Not to be confused with the infinitive **inculpate,** which means "to incriminate; accuse."

free from blame; guiltless; not culpable.

"Sometimes, **inculpable** defendants who are subjected to skillful cross-examination can be made to seem guilty of the crimes with which they are charged."

Related words: **inculpably** (in-KUL-pə-blee) *adverb;* **inculpability** (in-KUL-pə-BIL-i-tee) and **inculpableness** (in-KUL-pə-bəl-nis) *both nouns.*

indefatigable (IN-di-FAT-i-gə-bəl)

From Latin *indefatigabilis,* from *in-,* meaning "not," + *defatigare,* an infinitive meaning "to tire out, exhaust."

untiring; not yielding to fatigue; incapable of being worn out.

"Her **indefatigable** energy attracted many supporters to her cause, seeing in her capacity for hard work the solution to all their problems."

Related words: **indefatigably** (IN-di-FAT-i-gə-blee) *adverb;* **indefatigability** (IN-di-FAT-i-gə-BIL-i-tee) and **indefatigableness** (IN-di-FAT-i-gə-bəl-nis) *both nouns.*

indigenous (in-DIJ-ə-nəs)

From Latin adjective *indigen,* meaning "native"; from *gignere* an infinitive meaning "to beget, bear."

1. native to a country, a region, etc.

"Strangely, the **indigenous** population was never cruelly exploited by the invaders."

2. inborn; innate; natural.

"Despite the suggestions of certain anthropologists, nobody has offered acceptable proof that emotions are **indigenous** to all humans."

Related words: **indigenously** (in-DIJ-ə-nəs-lee) *adverb;* **indigenousness** (in-DIJ-ə-nəs-nis) *noun.*

indiscrete (IN-di-SKREET)

From Latin *indiscretus,* meaning "undivided."

Not to be confused with the universally understood **indiscreet** (same pronunciation), meaning "lacking good judgment." *See* **discrete.**

not divided into distinct parts; not detached, not discrete.

"To our chagrin, we found an **indiscrete** mass of miscellany that we would have to sort out."

indomitable (in-DOM-i-tə-bəl)
From Latin *indomitus,* meaning "untamed; ungovernable."

unconquerable; unyielding.

"All those present expressed admiration for the **indomitable** chief operating officer, who had accepted the challenge of working for a company about to go bankrupt and in a single year had turned it into a profitable enterprise."

Related words: **indomitably** (in-DOM-i-tə-blee) *adverb;* **indomitability** (in-DOM-i-tə-BIL-i-tee) and **indomitableness** (in-DOM-i-tə-bəl-nis) *both nouns.*

indurate (IN-duu-rit)
From Latin *induratus,* past participle of infinitive *indurare,* meaning "to harden."

callous; hardened; unfeeling.

"After careful consideration he came to the conclusion that Emily's **indurate** response had clearly been thought out, and there was nothing to do but abandon the possibility of marriage."

Related word: **induration** (IN-duu-RAY-shən) *noun.*

See also **obdurate.**

ineffable (in-EF-ə-bəl)
From Latin *ineffabilis,* meaning "unutterable," from *in-,* meaning "not," + *effabilis,* meaning "utterable."

And while there is the English word **effable,** meaning "utterable," you probably will seldom hear or read this word. At the same time, now that you have the word **ineffable,** be ready to hear it over and over again in years to come. Sometimes used without an understanding of what this popular word means.

unutterable; inexpressible; unspeakable.

"I was gripped by **ineffable** joy at hearing I would soon be given a promotion to a job worth doing."

Related words: **ineffably** (in-EF-ə-blee) *adverb*; **ineffability** (in-EF-ə-BIL-i-tee) and **ineffableness** (in-EF-ə-bəl-nis) *both nouns.*

ineluctable (IN-i-LUK-tə-bəl)

From Latin *ineluctabilis,* meaning "insurmountable," from *in-,* meaning "not," + *eluctari,* meaning "to surmount," + *-ible,* meaning "able."

inescapable; unavoidable.

"It appeared that an **ineluctable** force had him in its grip, and while he was certain he could never escape, he knew he had to continue struggling."

Related words: **ineluctably** (IN-i-LUK-tə-blee) *adverb*; **ineluctability** (IN-i-LUK-tə-BIL-ə-tee) *noun.*

inexorable (in-EK-sər-ə-bəl)

From Latin *inexorabilis,* meaning "incapable of being entreated."

unalterable; relentless; unyielding; unyielding to prayer or entreaty.

"He had been warned to stay away from banks that lend money too easily, and now he found out why—generous lenders at the drop of a hat had suddenly become **inexorable** creditors."

Related words: **inexorably** (in-EK-sər-ə-blee) *adverb*; **inexorability** (in-EK-sər-ə-BIL-ə-tee) and **inexorableness** (in-EK-sər-ə-bəl-nis) *both nouns.*

infrangible (in-FRAN-jə-bəl)

From Latin *infrangibilis,* meaning "unbreakable."

inviolable; which cannot be broken or infringed.

"She soon found out that the parietal rules at her new college were really intended to be **infrangible,** even though she considered them old-fashioned."

Related words: **infrangibly** (in-FRAN-jə-blee) *adverb*; **infrangibility** (in-FRAN-jə-BIL-i-tee) and **infrangibleness** (in-FRAN-jə-bəl-nis) *both nouns.*

ingenuous. *See* **disingenuous.**

inimitable (i-NIM-i-tə-bəl)

From Latin *inimitabilis,* meaning "incapable of imitation"; from *imitabilis,* meaning "imitable."

Far more successful as a negative word than the positive **imitable** (IM-i-tə-bəl), the implication being that while imitation may be thought to be the sincerest form of flattery, impossibility of imitation trumps the possibility of imitation.

unmatched; peerless; defying imitation.

"The family's **inimitable** skill on the high wire made the Wallendas the greatest circus attraction for generations."

Related words: **inimitably** (i-NIM-i-tə-blee) *adverb*; **inimitability** (i-NIM-i-tə-BIL-i-tee) and **inimitableness** (i-NIM-i-tə-bəl-nis) *both nouns*.

innocuous (i-NOK-yoo-əs)

From Latin *innocuus*, meaning "harmless," from Latin *in-*, meaning "not" + *noxius*, meaning "poisonous," whence came English **nocuous** (NOK-yoo-əs), meaning "poisonous," and **innocuous.**

harmless; not injurious; unlikely to offend.

"While the supervisor's **innocuous** remarks accomplished their overall purpose of giving offense to no one, they did little to instill confidence in her leadership."

Related words: **innocuously** (i-NOK-yoo-əs-lee) *adverb*; **innocuousness** (i-NOK-yoo-əs-nis) *noun*.

inordinate (in-OR-dn-it)

From Latin *inordinatus*, meaning "disordered, irregular."

excessive; not within proper limits; immoderate, uncontrolled.

"Everyone at the table noticed that during dinner the couple drank **inordinate** amounts of red wine."

Related words: **inordinately** (in-OR-dn-it-lee) *adverb*; **inordinateness** (in-OR-dn-it-nis) *noun*.

insalubrious (IN-sə-LOO-bree-əs)

From Latin *in-*, meaning "not," + *salubris*, meaning "health-giving, wholesome."

of climate, etc.: unwholesome; detrimental to health.

"In the tropics, where **insalubrious** nights follow sweltering days, the desire to work hard on his novel is easily defeated."

Related words: **insalubriously** (IN-sə-LOO-bree-əs-lee) *adverb*; **insalubrity** (IN-sə-LOO-bri-tee) *noun*.

insentient (in-SEN-shənt)

From English **in-**, meaning "not," + **sentient**, meaning "perceiving"; from Latin infinitive *sentire*, meaning "to feel."

inanimate; indifferent; destitute of physical feeling.

"What beauty and emotion the sculptor was capable of obtaining from **insentient** stone!"

Related words: **insentience** (in-SEN-shəns) and **insentiency** (in-SEN-shən-see) *both nouns.*

intemerate (in-TEM-ər-it)

From Latin *intemeratus*, meaning "unblemished"; from *in-*, meaning "not," + past participle of infinitive *temerare*, meaning "to violate."

Not to be confused with **intemperate** (in-TEM-pər-it), which deals most often with questions of a person's abstinence from booze but also with other questions of **temperament** (TEM-pər-ə-mənt), such as the ability to hold one's temper.

inviolable; undefiled; unblemished.

"The new senator was widely thought to be a lady of **intemerate** reputation and unsullied character, who would ably represent us in Washington."

Related words: **intemerately** (in-TEM-ər-it-lee) *adverb*; **intemerateness** (in-TEM-ər-it-nis) *noun.*

intemperate. *See* **intemerate.**

internecine (IN-tər-NEE-seen)

From Latin *internecinus*, meaning "murderous," from the infinitive verb *internecare*, meaning "to kill."

Can this etymology be your first clue to the fact that **internecine** says nothing of things happening *between* people or organizations? Forget for a moment the ordinary meanings of the Latin and English prefix *inter-* that you know so well. Especially forget the meaning "between peoples" that is often understood by the half educated.

Nevertheless, you are in good company when you consider that the person responsible for introducing and making respectable this misinformed idea was none other than Dr. Johnson himself, the idiosyncratic lexicographer who misdefined *internecine* as "endeavouring mutual destruction."

deadly; destructive; war to the death.

"Civilization has advanced to the point at which **internecine** warfare is considered successful when an opposing army is rendered less than fully effective, not when one side or the other is completely exterminated."

intestate (in-TES-tayt)

From Latin *intestatus*, from *in-*, meaning "not," + *testatus*, the past participle of *testari*, meaning "to bear witness; to make a will." *See also* **testate.**

1. of a person; not having made a will.

"The vain old man, without giving a thought to what would happen to his survivors, but happy that he could avoid letting anyone know how old he was, died **intestate.**"

2. of a thing: not disposed of by will; belonging to the estate of a person who dies without having made a will.

"Believe it or not, that woman's property was said to remain **intestate** for almost half a century after her death, and not a single heir has yet turned up."

intrepid. *See* trepid.

inveterate (in-VET-ər-it)

From Latin *inveteratus*, the past participle of verb *inveterare*, meaning "to grow old; preserve." *Inveteratus* is usually translated as "of long standing; inveterate."

chronic; habitual; long established; deep-rooted.

"By all accounts, Desmond has been an **inveterate** liar about his past and has never been confronted by anyone who knew the truth about him."

Related words: **inveterately** (in-VET-ər-it-lee) *adverb*; **inveterateness** (in-VET-ər-it-nis) *noun*.

invidious (in-VID-ee-əs)

From Latin *invidiosus*, meaning "envious; spiteful"; from *invidia*, meaning "envy; ill will."

1. obnoxious; intended to give offense.

"His special weakness after a few drinks is his propensity to make **invidious** comparisons that offend everyone within earshot."

2. injurious; tending to cause envy or resentment.

"Their father's **invidious** remarks unintentionally fed the siblings' long-festering rivalry."

Related words: **invidiously** (in-VID-ee-əs-lee) *adverb*; **invidious-ness** (in-VID-ee-əs-nis) *noun*.

invincible. *See* **vincible.**

irascible (i-RAS-ə-bəl)

From Latin *irascibilis*, from *irasci*, meaning "to grow angry."

irritable; hot-tempered; quick to anger.

"Eileen's wit and glib tongue did not lessen the sting of her **irascible** outbursts."

Related words: **irascibly** (i-RAS-ə-blee) *adverb*; **irascibility** (i-RAS-i-BIL-i-tee) and **irascibleness** (i-RAS-i-bəl-nis) *both nouns*.

irenic (i-REN-ik)

From Greek *eirenikós*, meaning "pacific; peaceful."

Also given as **irenical** (i-REN-i-kəl).

conciliatory; tending to promote peace or reconciliation.

"Much to our surprise, the most **irenic** elements in the government tended to be men who had spent their earlier careers as commanders in the military."

Related word: **irenically** (i-REN-i-klee) *adverb*.

iridescent. *See* **opalescent.**

irrefragable (i-REF-rə-gə-bəl)

From Latin *irrefragabilis*, from *ir-*, meaning "not," + infinitive *refragari*, meaning "to oppose, thwart," + -*bilis*, a suffix meaning "able."

incontestable; indisputable; incontrovertible.

"Soon we found that her arguments were **irrefragable,** and nothing could be gained by continuing the dispute."

Related words: **irrefragably** (i-REF-rə-gə-blee) *adverb*; **irrefragability** (i-REF-rə-gə-BIL-i-tee) and **irrefragableness** (i-REF-rə-gə-bəl-nis) *both nouns*.

irrefrangible (IR-i-FRAN-jə-bəl)

From English **ir-**, meaning "not," + **frangible**, meaning "breakable," from the Latin infinitive *frangere*, meaning "to break."

A verb form of special interest because its past participle *fractum* gives us the Engish word *fracture*.

inviolable; not to be violated; not to be broken.

"For a school that claims to be entirely open and relaxed in its discipline, Excelsior Prep enforces a great number of **irrefrangible** regulations."

Related words: **irrefrangibly** (IR-i-FRAN-jə-blee) *adverb*; **irrefrangibility** (IR-i-FRAN-jə-BIL-i-tee) and **irrefrangibleness** (IR-i-FRAN-jə-bəl-nis) *both nouns.*

ithyphallic (ITH-ə-FAL-ik)

From Latin *ithyphallicus*, from Greek *ithyphallikós* from *ithy*, meaning "straight or erect," + *phallós*, meaning "phallus," + *-ikos*, having the same meaning as the English suffix *-ic*.

Although **ithyphallic** has denotations concerned with festivals of the ancient god Bacchus, one of whose titles was that of god of wine, the emphasis here is on a modern meaning of this term. Yet we must recognize that statues of Bacchus portrayed him as a man with enviably ramrod intensity.

grossly indecent; obscene.

"A Supreme Court justice is reputed to have said of **ithyphallic** writing, 'I can't define it but I know it when I see it.'"

J

jackbooted (JAK-BOO-tid)

Straight out of the Harley-Davidson popular image: from English **jackboot,** meaning "a popular style of leather boot," + a suffix signifying a past participle, **-ed.**

1. wearing jackboots, especially said of those who ride motorcycles.

"When the **jackbooted** crowd roared into town, women gripped their purses tighter and ordinary men did their best to find shelter without allowing themselves to appear frightened."

2. characterized by rough, bullying tactics.

"The diner was suddenly crowded with **jackbooted,** tattooed, hirsute men."

Janus-faced (JAY-nəs-FAYST)

From the name of the ancient god Janus, a two-faced personage, who was in charge of guarding the gates to heaven. His extraordinary number of faces was of special interest.

1. two-faced; deceitful.

"If you had listened carefully to what the **Janus-faced** supervisor was saying, you would have known he was the treacherous man we all had to fear."

2. having one face looking ahead, the other looking other backward.

"Most historical accounts I have read seem **Janus-faced,** more interested in making judgments on the events of the twentieth century than predictions on the twenty-first."

jaundiced (JAWN-dist)

> From English **jaundice**, from Old French *jaunisse*, from Latin *galbinus*, all meaning "greenish yellow."

> 1. showing prejudice, as from envy, etc.

> "We distrusted her judgment of her colleagues, knowing as we did that she regarded them with a **jaundiced** eye."

> 2. affected with jaundice.

> "The young physician immediately suspected that I was **jaundiced** when he saw my yellow skin."

jejune (ji-JOON)

> From Latin *ieiunus*, meaning "fasting; hungry; meager; feeble."

> 1. dull, insipid; juvenile, immature.

> "His maundering conversation was surprisingly **jejune** for someone who held such an important position."

> 2. of a diet: lacking in nutritive value.

> "I fear the children are malnourished on the **jejune** diet they are receiving."

> Related words: **jejunely** (ji-JOON-lee) *adverb*; **jejuneness** (ji-JOON-nis) and **jejunity** (ji-JOON-ni-tee) *both nouns*.

jiggered (JIG-ərd)

> Colloquial, origin unknown.

> exhausted; damned; devitalized.

> "At the disappointing news, the poor man spat out, 'I'll be **jiggered**,' and fell silent, apparently feeling better because he had taken a load off his mind."

jocose (joh-KOHS)

> From Latin *iocus*, meaning "joking," + *-osus*, meaning "full of."

> of persons or activities: given to joking or jesting; playful; sportive.

> "The games were accompanied by much **jocose** banter occasioned particularly by our host's social pretensions."

> Related words: **jocosely** (joh-KOHS-lee) *adverb*; **jocoseness** (joh-KOHS-nis) and **jocosity** (joh-KOS-i-tee) *both nouns*.

jocular (JOK-yə-lər)

> From Latin *iocularis*, meaning "little joke," from *iocus*, meaning "joke," + *-ulus*, a diminutive suffix.

> given to joking or jesting.

"She made the error of submitting as her first paper a short piece sprinkled with inappropriately **jocular** remarks."

Related words: **jocularly** (JOK-yə-lər-lee) *adverb*; **jocularity** (JOK-yə-LAR-i-tee) *noun.*

jocund (JOK-ənd)

From Latin *iocundus* or *iucundus,* meaning "pleasant"; from the infinitive *iuvare,* meaning "to assist," + *-cundus,* an adjectival suffix.

merry; blithe; glad.

"The seriousness of the situation was leavened by his *jocund* repartee, which never stopped for a moment."

Related words: **jocundly** (JOK-ənd-lee) *adverb*; **jocundity** (joh-KUND-i-tee) *noun.*

judicable (JOO-di-kə-bəl)

From Late Latin *iudicabilis,* from infinitive *iudicare,* meaning "to judge," + *-abilis,* a suffix meaning "able."

capable of being judged; liable to judgment.

"In the judgment of the Queen's Counsel, the question is only marginally **judicable** and, therefore, should not be taken up in the courts."

judicious (joo-DISH-əs)

From French *judicieux* and Italian *giudizioso,* both from Latin *iudictum,* meaning "judgment."

wise; exercising sound judgment.

"By **judicious** apportionment of your time, one-half for study of your three courses and the other half for the major examinations you will face in two months, you will surely be able to handle the demands put upon you."

Related words: **judiciously** (joo-DISH-əs-lee) *adverb*; **judiciousness** (joo-DISH-əs-nis) *noun.*

juridical (juu-RID-i-kəl)

From Latin *juridicialis,* meaning "of law, juridical."

Also given as **juridic** (juu-RID-ik).

relating to the administration of law or judicial proceedings.

"I have learned much of **juridical** ins and outs from watching *Law and Order* and other TV shows relating to the law."

Related word: **juridically** (juu-RID-i-kəl-ee) *adverb.*

juvenescent (JOO-və-NES-ənt)

From Latin *iuvenescens*, present participle of infinitive *iuvenescere*, meaning "to become youthful."

growing young or youthful.

"The old man decided to give up tennis at his club, because his erstwhile partners were discouragingly **juvenescent** and never tired of chasing balls he could not reach."

Related word: **juvenescence** (JOO-və-NES-əns) *noun.*

K

Kafkaesque (KAHF-kə-ESK)
From the name of Franz Kafka (1883–1924), an Austrian novelist and short-story writer.

suggesting a nightmarish or illogical quality to events; resembling the literary work of Kafka.

"Imagine a **Kafkaesque** situation in which a person who may either be innocent or guilty of a crime is imprisoned and interrogated endlessly by police without knowing what crime the police have in mind."

kaput (kah-PUUT)
Slang. From German *kaputt*, from French *(être) capot*, meaning "(to be) trickless in the game of piquet" and, therefore, "ruined."

ruined; unable to continue; bankrupt.

"Many of the companies whose stock prices soared in the late '90s were **kaput** in the new millennium."

kempt (kempt)
From Old English *cemb* (also spelled many other ways), past participle of infinitive *cemban*, meaning "to comb."

One of those words that have been written off as archaic many times in their thousand years of life but are still kicking. How it holds up against the competition of **unkempt** (un-KEMPT) is not known for certain. After all, people who comb their hair just now and then far outnumber those who do so regularly.

of a home: neat; tidy; of someone's hair: combed.

"When we consider that electricity was far from a reality in the coal mining villages of an earlier century, we must wonder how housewives were able to keep their homes **kempt** and their many children's hair washed and untangled."

kittenish (KIT-n-ish)

From the English familiar word **kitten** + **-ish,** an adjectival suffix meaning "like."

playful; like a kitten.

"Away from the watchful eye of her grandmother, Gigi became irrepressibly **kittenish**."

Related words: **kittenishly** (KIT-n-ish-lee) *adverb*; **kittenishness** (KIT-n-ish-nis) *noun.*

kleptomaniac (KLEP-tə-MAY-nee-AK)

From English **kleptomania** (KLEP-tə-MAY-nee-ə), from Greek *klepto,* a combining form of *kléptes,* meaning "thief," + the familiar *mania.*

Also given as **cleptomaniac** (same pronunciation).

If one examines words originally used to describe what our modern intelligentsia consider mental diseases, we would find quite a few with *-mania* and *-maniac* imbedded in them—consider "dipsomania" and "dipsomaniac." How prescient, how mistaken we were!

pertaining to a person who is described as having an irresistible urge to steal.

"Our townspeople learned to pity and tolerate **kleptomaniac** behavior when they realized how compulsive it was."

Related word: **kleptomania** (KLEP-tə-MAY-nee-ə) *noun.*

klutzy (KLUT-see)

American slang, from Yiddish *klots,* literally "a wooden block," + *-y,* a suffix meaning "inclined to."

awkward, clumsy; socially inept; foolish.

"The **klutzy** ladies of the back line in a cheap burlesque house were not thought of as dancers, but as overweight sex objects."

Related words: **klutz** (kluts) and **klutziness** (KLUT-see-nis) *both nouns.*

knurled (nurld)

Possibly from Middle English *knorre,* meaning "a knot," + *-ed,* an adjectival suffix.

of a knob, etc.: having small ridges on a surface.

"Without the **knurled** edge, neither my wife nor I would ever have been able to open a jar of martini onions."

Related words: **knur** (nur) and **knurling** (NUR-ling) *both nouns;* **knurly** (NUR-lee) *adjective.*

L

labyrinthine (LAB-ə-RIN-thin)

    From English **labyrinth**, meaning "a maze," + **-ine**, an adjectival suffix meaning "like." From Latin *labyrinthus*, from Greek *labyrinthós*, both meaning "labyrinth or maze."

    Also given as **labyrinthian** (LAB-ə-RIN-thee-ən).

    1. of the nature of a maze.

        "We would not have built an interesting, **labyrinthine** kitchen if we had known you cooked only occasionally and didn't mind getting lost in your own home."

    2. intricate; complicated; involved.

        "I tried hard but could scarcely follow his endless **labyrinthine** sentences, with here and there an interesting word or phrase incorporated to sustain my interest."

    Related words: **labyrinth** (LAB-ə-rinth) *noun*; **labyrinthic** (LAB-ə-RIN-thik) *adjective*; **labyrinthically** (LAB-ə-RIN-thi-kə-lee) *adverb*.

lachrymose (LAK-rə-MOHS)

    From Latin *lacrimosus*, meaning "tearful, lamentable"; from *lacrima*, meaning "a tear," + *-osus*, an adjectival suffix meaning "given to."

    1. mournful; given to shedding tears.

        "The sentimental film evoked a **lachrymose** response from the impressionable young girls."

    2. tearful; tending to provoke tears.

        "The child actress was amazingly adept at delivering a **lachrymose** performance at will."

Related words: **lachrymosely** (LAK-rə-MOHS-lee) *adverb*; **lachrymosity** (LAK-rə-MOS-i-tee) *noun*.

laconic (lə-KON-ik)

From Latin *Laconicus*, from Greek *Lakonikós*, both meaning "a Laconian"—a Spartan—ancient Sparta having been the capital of Laconia.

And, of course, Laconians were famous for their **laconic**—brusque and aphoristic—speech, as were the Spartans for their courage, frugality, and stern discipline.

in speech and writing: concise, brief, and crammed with wisdom.

"What my boss expects most are **laconic** replies to his questions, but they must be written, not spoken, and be submitted quickly."

Related words: **laconically** (lə-KON-ik-ə-lee) *adverb*; **laconism** (LAK-ə-NIZ-əm) *noun*.

lambent (LAM-bənt)

From Latin *lambens*, present participle of *lambere*, meaning "to wash, to lick."

1. of light or fire: playing lightly over a surface.

"The coals had long been gray, but **lambent** tongues of flame continued to dance over the embers occasionally."

2. of wit, style, etc.: playing lightly or brilliantly over its subject.

"Once again, with his **lambent** wit and good humor, M. DeBeauvivier managed to entice his students into working on a difficult project that would teach them something that excited them intellectually."

Related words: **lambently** (LAM-bənt-lee) *adverb*; **lambency** (LAM-bən-see) *noun*.

languid (LANG-gwid)

From Latin *languidus*, meaning "faint, sluggish," from *languere*, meaning "to languish."

1. wanting in vigor or vitality.

"It was obvious that his recent illness had left him **languid** and weak."

2. apathetic; showing little interest or concern.

"I could tell from his **languid** attitude he had little chance to survive his initial interview, much less the entire series of meetings we normally scheduled."

Related words: **languidly** (LANG-gwid-lee) *adverb*; **languidness** (LANG-gwid-nis) *noun*; **languishing** (LANG-gwi-shing) *adjective*.

See also **languorous**.

languorous (LANG-gər-əs)

From English **languor**, meaning "sluggishness," + -**ous** "full of"; from Middle English *langour* "sickness"; from Latin infinitive *languere*, meaning "to languish."

inducing lassitude or weakness; languid.

"A torpor came over him, a **languorous** inability to rouse himself from the apathy that was beginning to grip him and would soon have him in its clutches."

Related words: **languorously** (LANG-gər-əs-lee) *adverb*; **languorousness** (LANG-gər-eus-nis) *noun*.

lanuginose (lə-NOO-jə-NOHS)

From Latin *lanuginosus*, meaning "downy," from *lanugo*, meaning "wooliness," + -*osus*, an adjectival suffix meaning "abounding in."

Also given as **lanuginous** (lə-NOO-jə-nəs).

downy; covered with soft down.

"Where we had expected to find a scaly outer skin, we were surprised to find the creature had a **lanuginose** covering from neck to tail."

Related words: **lanugo** (lə-NOO-goh) and **lanuginousness** (lə-NOO-jə-nəs-nis) *both nouns*.

Laodicean (lay-OD-ə-SEE-ən)

From Laodicea, the ancient name of Latakia, Syria, whose inhabitants were said to care little about Christianity.

in religious or political beliefs: indifferent; lukewarm.

"Anne told me her entire family maintained a **Laodicean** attitude toward matters of churchgoing and other religious observances, thus absolving them of the guilt associated with neglect of duties toward God."

lascivious (lə-SIV-ee-əs)

From Latin *lascivia*, meaning "playfulness, impudence, lewdness."

1. wanton; inclined to lust.

"The boy, scarcely more than ten years old, was reported by his classmates to have made **lascivious** gestures and remarks."

2. arousing; inciting to lust.

> "Some of the photographs of undraped figures were considered **lascivious**, and the photographer was asked to eliminate them from the exhibit."

Related words: **lasciviously** (lə-SIV-ee-əs-lee) *adverb*; **lasciviousness** (lə-SIV-ee-əs-nis) *noun*.

laudable (LAW-də-bəl)

From Latin *laudabilis*, meaning "praiseworthy"; from infinitive *laudare*, meaning "to praise."

of things and actions: commendable; deserving praise.

> "The judges were nearly unanimous in finding the neophyte composer's works **laudable** in form and originality."

Related words: **laudably** (LAW-də-blee) *adverb*; **laudableness** (LAW-də-bəl-nis), **laudability** (LAW-də-BIL-i-tee), and **laudation** (law-DAY-shən) *all nouns*.

See **laudatory**.

laudatory (LAW-də-TOR-ee)

From Latin *laudatorius*, meaning "expressive of praise"; from the infinitive *laudare*, meaning "to praise."

Also given as **laudative** (LAW-də-tiv). *See also* **laudable**.

eulogistic; expressing or containing praise.

> "I soon found it quite easy to give a **laudatory** speech introducing my friend, as he is a man I much admire."

Related word: **laudatorily** (LAW-də-TOR-i-lee) *adverb*.

leonine (LEE-ə-NĪN)

From Latin *leoninus*, meaning "lionlike."

lionlike; resembling or suggestive of a lion.

> "The old senator with his **leonine** appearance and booming voice easily commanded the attention of Washington reporters and members of the House of Representatives."

libidinous (li-BID-n-əs)

From Latin *libidinosis*, meaning "willful, arbitrary; sensual, lustful"; from *libido*, meaning "lust," + *-osus*, meaning "full of."

Also given as **libidinal** (li-BID-n-əl).

lustful, lewd, lecherous, lascivious.

"An elderly, **libidinous** gentleman these days is often referred to as a dirty old man."

Related words: **libido** (li-BEE-doh) and **libidinousness** (li-BID-n-əs-nis) *both nouns*; **libidinally** (li-BID-n-ə-lee) and **libidinously** (li-BID-n-əs-lee) *both adverbs*.

licentious (lī-SEN-shəs)

From Latin *licentiosus*, meaning "unrestrained," from *licentia*, meaning "license."

sexually unrestrained; immoral, lawless; lascivious, libertine.

"Greek-letter fraternities on some campuses provide beer, whiskey, food, women, and venues for **licentious** parties."

Related words: **licentiously** (lī-SEN-shəs-lee) *adverb*; **licentiousness** (lī-SEN-shəs-nis) *noun*.

licit (LIS-it)

From Latin *licitus*, meaning "lawful," past participle of infinitive *licere*, meaning "it is permitted or it is lawful."

allowable, permissible; lawful.

"People being what they are, the adjective **illicit** is far better known than **licit,** and far more useful."

Related word: **licitly** (LIS-it-lee) *adverb*.

light-fingered (LĪT-FING-gərd)

From well-known English **light**, and **fingered**, meaning "having fingers."

thieving; skilled at picking pockets and shoplifting.

"We usually would remember to lock the silver when my father's **light-fingered** associate came to the house."

Related word: **light-fingeredness** (LĪT-FING-gərd-nis) noun.

Lilliputian (LIL-i-PYOO-shən)

From *Lilliput*, the name of the tiny people of an imaginary country in Jonathan Swift's *Gulliver's Travels*.

1. of persons: diminutive, extremely small.

"It did not enter her mind for a moment that her **Lilliputian** husband-to-be was at least six inches shorter than she."

2. of worldly matters: petty; trivial.

"When Joan finally had time to stop and think, she realized her portion of the estate was **Lilliputian** and might pay for a month's supply of first-class postage stamps."

lily-livered (LIL-ee-LIV-ərd)

From well-known English **lily** and **liver** + **-ed,** enabling **livered** to function as a past participle.

An old superstition had it that a coward's liver contained no blood, so a person said to be cowardly was considered **lily-livered.**

pusillanimous; lacking in courage.

"Most people were afraid of me when I was a young man, but I knew I was **lily-livered** and was grateful that no one challenged me."

limpid (LIM-pid)

From Latin *limpidus*, meaning "clear." One of those wonderful words telling us everything is A-OK.

1. of liquid: transparent, clear, pellucid.

"Julian's martinis were as **limpid** and cold as an alpine stream."

2. of writing: lucid, free from obscurity.

"I admired his **limpid** writing, which clarified the most abstruse problems."

3. of emotion: free from worry, completely calm.

"What she really longed for was a **limpid** existence, a life moving seamlessly from day to day without fear of interruption."

Related words: **limpidly** (LIM-pid-lee) *adverb*; **limpidness** (LIM-pid-nis) and **limpidity** (lim-PID-i-tee) *both nouns.*

lissome (LIS-əm)

Possibly a contracted form of the adjective **lithesome,** reflecting a linguistic practice of the British. After all, the British taught us to pronounce the name Worcester as though it were written Wooster. And now, at least in the United States, we have places named Wooster and at least one college by that name.

So **lissome** seems to have become a spelling of **lithesome,** and both terms came from the German *lind*, meaning "mild," and from the Latin *lentus*, meaning "slow."

Also given as **lissom,** with the same pronunciation.

lithe; flexible; supple; agile.

"The leopard's **lissome** gait astonished all who had never before seen the animal in hot pursuit of game."

Related words: **lissomely** (LIS-əm-lee) *adverb*; **lissomeness** (LIS-əm-nis) *noun*.

litigious (li-TIJ-əs)

From Latin *litigiosus*, meaning "quarrelsome, contentious," from *litigium*, meaning "a quarrel."

1. contentious; inclined readily to sue.

"After serving a year's apprenticeship in a **litigious** New York firm, Spencer found himself unable to adjust to the relaxed practice of law in the Maine backwoods where he chose to live."

2. pertaining to lawsuits or litigation.

"The young attorney's **litigious** experience is far from adequate to consider asking him to see their case through."

Related words: **litigiously** (li-TIJ-əs-lee) *adverb*; **litigiousness** (li-TIJ-əs-nis) and **litigiosity** (li-TIJ-ee-OS-i-tee) *both nouns*.

littoral (LIT-ər-əl)

From Latin *littoralis* or *litoralis*, meaning "of the shore," from *litus*, meaning "shore, coast, bank."

pertaining to the shore or beach, etc., of a body of water.

"Rich colonies of **littoral** bivalves once found along the Erie are rarely seen today because of the large vessels on the lake and the many thriving industries long established there."

liverish (LIV-ər-ish)

From English **liver**, "a bodily organ" + **-ish**, an adjectival suffix meaning "like."

A function of the **liver**, once thought to be the seat of love, is to purify the blood, a vital function.

1. disagreeable, melancholy.

"It once was common for a **liverish** person to blame the uncontrollable malfunctioning of his bodily organs for the way he behaved."

2. bilious; having a liver disorder.

"My oldest uncle found it convenient to complain of being **liverish** when all he had to do was stop eating and drinking so much."

loathsome (LOH*TH*-səm)

From Middle English *lothsom* from *loth* or *lath*, meaning "evil," + the adjectival suffix *-some*.

repulsive; causing disgust or loathing; hateful, odious, shocking.

"The skin condition that plagued him was a **loathsome** case of psoriasis, which often made it necessary for him to be hospitalized."

Related words: **loathsomely** (LOH*TH*-səm-lee) *adverb*; **loathsomeness** (LOH*TH*-səm-nis) *noun*.

loquacious (loh-KWAY-shəs)

From English noun **loquacity**, meaning "talkativeness," + **-ous,** "given to"; from Latin *loquax*, meaning "talkative, chattering"; from the Latin infinitive *loqui*, meaning "to talk."

garrulous; talkative; chattering, babbling.

"Our **loquacious** neighbor cast a pall over the party, with her inane chatter stifling any attempt to start an interesting conversation."

Related words: **loquaciously** (loh-KWAY-shəs-lee) *adverb*; **loquaciousness** (loh-KWAY-shəs-nis) and **loquacity** (loh-KWAS-i-tee) *both nouns.*

louche (loosh)

From French *louche*, meaning "squinting," from Latin *luscus*, meaning "one-eyed."

oblique, not straightforward; shady, disreputable.

"There was something **louche** about the caretaker we had recently hired, and we regretted having entrusted our house keys to him."

lubricious (loo-BRISH-əs)

From English **lubric,** an archaic word meaning "shifty," + *-ious*, meaning "characteristically."

Also given as **lubricous** (LOO-bri-kəs), not used much.

slippery, smooth; slimy, oily; lustful, lecherous.

"Not often do we find a **lubricious** person who proves eventually to be upstanding and trustworthy."

Related words: **lubriciously** (loo-BRISH-əs-lee) *adverb*; **lubricity** (loo-BRIS-i-tee) *noun*.

luculent (LOO-kyuu-lənt)

From Latin *luculentus*, meaning "bright, brilliant, rich"; from *lux*, meaning "light," + *-ulentus*, a Latin adjectival suffix meaning "full of," translated into English as **-ulent** with the same meaning, for example, as in **flatulent.**

1. lucid; clear.

"Above all, his ability to write **luculent** prose brought him to the attention of the army command."

2. convincing, pertinent.

"The **luculent** argument she presented to the jury in her summary was the best oration I have ever heard her give."

Related word: **luculently** (LUU-kyuu-lənt-lee) *adverb.*

Lucullan (loo-KUL-ən)

From the Roman name *Lucullus,* known principally as the name of a wealthy ancient general and administrator who liked his food and spared no expense in entertaining.

In Lucullus's later years food became the center of his life. It was said that even when he dined alone his table was superb, and he left his mark in the sentence "Lucullus will sup tonight with Lucullus," which has become the trademark of a glutton who eats alone.

Lucullan is given also as **Lucullean** and as **Lucullian** (both pronounced LOO-kə-LEE-ən).

of banquets and the like: sumptuous.

"Once Edgar became head of his company he achieved fame for the **Lucullan** feasts he provided for his numerous guests at his monthly first-Thursday-night galas."

lugubrious (luu-GOO-bree-əs)

From Latin *lugubris,* meaning "mournful."

exaggeratedly doleful, mournful, sorrowful.

"He wanted to relieve the oppressiveness of the **lugubrious** occasion by leaving instructions for those who would be called on to speak at his funeral to tell funny stories about his life."

Related words: **lugubriously** (luu-GOO-bree-əs-lee) *adverb*; **lugubriousness** (luu-GOO-bree-əs-nis) and **lugubriosity** (lə-GOO-bree-OS-i-tee) *both nouns.*

lupine (LOO-pīn)

From Latin *lupinus,* meaning "of a wolf."

having the qualities of a wolf; savage; predatory.

"An inexperienced person trying to make her way in Hollywood on her own might find the motion picture way of doing business **lupine,** to say the least."

Not to be confused with the plant called **lupine** (LOO-pin)—notice the difference in pronunciation—whose name also derives from *lupinus,* originally perhaps a German word, *Wolfsbohne,* literally "wolf bean."

lurid (LUUR-id)

From Latin *luridus,* meaning "pale yellow, ghastly, wan."

1. revolting; horrible, gruesome.

"I don't know why Jon insists on relating all the **lurid** details of everything he reads about in the tabloid newspapers."

2. shocking; ghastly, ominous.

"I have had enough of the **lurid** tales complete with mangled corpses and noisy gunfire that occupy moviemakers and television shows night after night."

Related words: **luridly** (LOO-rid-lee) *adverb;* **luridness** (LOO-rid-nis) *noun.*

M

Machiavellian (MAK-ee-ə-VEL-ee-ən)

From the name of Niccolò Machiavelli (1469–1527), the celebrated Florentinian statesman and author of *Il principe (The Prince)*, on the art of government. To his surname is added the adjectival suffix *-ian*, meaning "characteristic of."

Also given as **Machiavelian** (same pronunciation).

astute; practicing duplicity in statecraft or in general conduct.

"Cynicism has become so widespread that many persons attribute **Machiavellian** motives to leaders in all walks of life."

Related word: **Machiavellianly** (MAK-ee-ə-VEL-ee-ən-lee) *adverb.*

macroscopic (MAK-rə-SKOP-ik)

From English **macro** "large" + **-scope**, a combining form meaning "instrument for viewing" + **-ic**, an adjectival suffix meaning "like."

Also given as **macroscopical** (MAK-rə-SKOP-ik-əl).

visible to the unassisted eye.

"The pathologist explained that after she conducts a **macroscopic** examination of the corpse to obtain an overall impression, it is her practice to then conduct a **microscopic** examination of tissues from the damaged portions of the body."

Related word: **macroscopically** (MAK-rə-SKOP-ik-ə-lee) *adverb.*

maculate (MAK-yə-lit)

From Latin *maculatus*, meaning "stained, defiled"; past participle of infinitive *maculare*, meaning "to stain, defile."

It speaks well of us universally that we far better know the adjective **immaculate** (i-MAK-yə-lit), which means "spotlessly clean," even as we eschew the term in describing our own behavior or reputations.

stained, spotted.

> "Her unfortunately **maculate** record in mathematics fresh in her mind, the poor sophomore wondered whether she could keep the rest of her grades high enough to compete for a good scholarship against her brilliant classmates."

Related words: **macula** (MAK-yə-lə) and **maculation** (MAK-yə-LAY-shən) *both nouns.*

magnanimous (mag-NAN-ə-məs)
From Latin *magnanimus*, meaning "great, brave"; from Latin *magnus*, meaning "great," + *animus*, meaning "mind, soul."

1. generously forgiving; free of vindictiveness.

> "The losing candidate was entirely **magnanimous** in immediately acknowledging defeat at the hands of the challenger."

2. noble in conduct; high-minded.

> "His contemporaries considered their leader a kind and **magnanimous** ruler who would ensure that all citizens are given fair treatment."

Related words: **magnanimously** (mag-NAN-ə-məs-lee) *adverb*; **magnanimousness** (mag-NAN-ə-məs-nis) and **magnanimity** (MAG-nə-NIM-i-tee) *both nouns.*

magniloquent (mag-NIL-ə-kwənt)
From Latin *magniloquus*, meaning "boastful."

bombastic; pompous; ambitious in expression.

> "We had been led to believe he was a stimulating speaker and were disappointed to find he was nothing but a **magniloquent** bore."

Related words: **magniloquently** (mag-NIL-ə-kwənt-lee) *adverb*; **magniloquence** (mag-NIL-ə-kwəns) *noun.*

majuscule. *See* **minuscule.**

maladroit (MAL-ə-DROYT)
From French *maladroit*, meaning "clumsy, awkward."

Fortunately, we also have the frequently used word **adroit** (ə-DROYT) with meanings opposite to those of **maladroit.**

awkward; bungling; tactless.

"Benjamin is a disaster at parties, **adroit** at putting his foot into his mouth whenever he speaks and **maladroit** on the dance floor, as though dancing with two left feet."

Related words: **maladroitly** (MAL-ə-DROYT-lee) *adverb*; **maladroitness** (MAL-ə-DROYT-nis) *noun*.

malapropos (MAL-ap-rə-POH)
From French *mal à propos*, meaning "inopportune," literally "badly (suited) to the purpose."

inappropriate; inopportune.

"Sara had a knack for choosing **malapropos** moments for asking personal questions."

malevolent (mə-LEV-ə-lənt)
From Latin *malevolens*, meaning "spiteful"; from the combining form *male*, meaning "evil," + *volens*, the present participle of the infinitive *velle*, meaning "to want or desire."

wishing evil to others; evil, injurious.

"I find it mystifying that an otherwise pleasant person can harbor such **malevolent** intentions toward anyone he has just met."

Related words: **malevolently** (mə-LEV-ə-lənt-lee) *adverb*; **malevolence** (mə-LEV-ə-ləns) *noun*.

malodorous (mal-OH-dər-əs)
From English **mal-,** a combining form meaning "bad," + **odorous,** meaning "yielding an odor."

evil smelling; having an unpleasant odor.

"At the general election, voters made it clear they did not want the **malodorous** pig farms anywhere near their town."

Related words: **malodorously** (mal-OH-dər-əs-lee) *adverb*; **malodor** (mal-OH-dər) and **malodorousness** (mal-OH-dər-əs-nis) *both nouns*.

marmoreal (mahr-MOR-ee-əl)
From Latin *marmoreus*, meaning "of marble, like marble"; from Greek *mármaros*, meaning "marble."

Also given as **marmorean** (mahr-MOR-ee-ən).

made of or like marble.

"After we enjoyed the **marmoreal** pleasures of the Greek galleries, we sampled the armoreal offerings of the medieval rooms."

Related word: **marmoreally** (mahr-MOR-ee-ə-lee) *adverb.*

matutinal (mə-TOOT-n-l)

From Latin *matutinalis,* meaning "early, of the morning"; from *matutinus,* meaning "of the morning," after *Matuta,* goddess of dawn.

early; performed in the morning.

"Without being asked, the young boy performed his **matutinal** chores of taking out garbage and putting clean dishes on their shelves."

Related word: **matutinally** (mə-TOOT-n-ə-lee) *adverb.*

maudlin (MAWD-lin)

From a variant form of the name Mary Magdalene—in Latin and in Greek, of course—a penitent whose eyes were often represented in art as swollen from weeping.

foolishly sentimental: mawkishly emotional.

"He managed to keep body and soul together by writing **maudlin** stories about little boys and girls deserted by their parents and forced to find their own way through life."

Related words: **maudlinly** (MAWD-lin-lee) *adverb;* **maudlinness** (MAWD-lin-nis) and **maudlinism** (MAWD-lin-iz-m) *both nouns.*

mediocre (MEE-dee-OH-kər)

From Latin *mediocris,* meaning "middling, average; at middling height."

of indifferent qualities; neither good nor bad, talented or untalented, etc.

"Meagan seemed to be content with doing **mediocre** work, never extending herself to her capability."

Related word: **mediocrity** (MEE-dee-OK-ri-tee) *noun.*

mellifluous (mə-LIF-loo-əs)

From Latin *mellifluus,* from *mel,* meaning "honey," + the infinitive *fluere,* meaning "to flow," + *-us,* an adjectival suffix meaning "full of."

Also given as **mellifluent** (mə-LIF-loo-ənt) with the same English meaning given below.

sweet as honey; sweet-sounding; smoothly flowing.

"We were transported by the sweet sound of the soprano's **mellifluous** voice."

Related words: **mellifluously** (mə-LIF-loo-əs-lee) *adverb*; **mellifluousness** (mə-LIF-loo-əs-nis) *noun*.

mendacious (men-DAY-shəs)

From Latin *mendax*, meaning "lying, deceiving," + -*ous*, an adjectival suffix meaning "full of."

telling lies; untruthful; false.

"When I found out that my **mendacious** cousin was the source of the rumor, I was hurt and angry."

Related words: **mendaciously** (men-DAY-shəs-lee) *adverb*; **mendaciousness** (men-DAY-shəs-nis) and **mendacity** (men-DAS-i-tee) *both nouns*.

mephitic (mə-FIT-ik)

From Latin *mephiticus*, an adjectival form of the noun *mephitis*, which means "noxious vapor."

From the accounts of an ancient people who sought protection against such vapors sent from a goddess in charge of the pertinent phenomena. Truly understandable. Well into modern times it was thought the disease called malaria was caused by vapors arising from the earth in swampy areas.

noxious; poisonous, pestilential; offensive to the smell.

"The **mephitic** fumes in the air-conditioned laboratory alerted us to a big problem."

Related words: **mephitically** (mə-FIT-ik-əl-ee) *adverb*; **mephitis** (mə-FĪ-tis) *noun*.

meretricious (MER-i-TRISH-əs)

From Latin *meretricius*, meaning "of a prostitute"; from infinitive *merere*, meaning "to earn money"—which may help us look differently at the economic role of prostitutes.

1. tawdry: flashy, vulgarly attractive.

"In spite of the **meretricious** gaudiness of Las Vegas, I must admit it was amusing and interesting for its half-dressed show girls."

2. pretentious, insincere.

"The **meretricious** ceremonies that accompanied his elevation to the presidency seemed entirely inappropriate for a democracy."

3. characteristic of a prostitute.

"Her father told her the clothing and makeup she wore appeared **meretricious** and to go to her room and not come back until she looked more respectable."

Related words: **meretriciously** (MER-i-TRISH-əs-lee) *adverb*; **meretriciousness** (MER-i-TRISH-əs-nis) *noun*.

mettlesome (MET-l-səm)

From English **mettle**, meaning "courage," + **-some**, an adjectival suffix.

of persons or animals: courageous; spirited.

"A **mettlesome** Olympic runner suddenly appeared to leave the pack and move almost effortlessly into the lead, never to be caught again by the others."

microscopic. *See* **macroscopic.**

mimetic (mi-MET-ik)

From Greek *mimetikós*, meaning "imitative" from *mímesis*, meaning "imitation"; giving us the English noun **mimesis** (mi-MEE-sis), meaning "imitation" or "mimicry."

characterized by the nature of imitation or mimicry.

"**Mimetic** primates readily learn to imitate repeated movements by their handlers and can mistakenly be thought to be in communication with them."

Related words: **mimetism** (MIM-i-TIZ-əm) *noun*; **mimetically** (mi-MET-i-kə-lee) *adverb*.

minacious (mi-NAY-shəs)

From Latin *minax*, meaning "overhanging," + *-ius*, an adjectival suffix.

Also given as **minatory** (MIN-ə-TOR-ee) and **minatorial** (MIN-ə-TOR-ee-əl), meaning "threatening."

menacing, threatening; full of threats.

"Implicit in the diplomat's words was a clearly **minacious** message to the effect that our country would respond immediately if missiles were launched at any of our friends."

Related words: **minaciously** (mi-NAY-shəs-lee) and **minatorily**

(MIN-ə-TOR-i-lee) *both adverbs;* **minaciousness** (mi-NAY-shəs-nis) and **minacity** (mi-NAS-i-tee) *both nouns.*

minatory. *See* **minacious.**

mingy (MIN-jee)
From English **m(ean)** and **(st)ingy,** "mean and stingy."

disappointingly small; niggardly, mean, stingy.

"Whoever designed my electronic wristwatch forgot that almost every adult has fingers that are too large to handle the **mingy** controls."

minuscule (MIN-ə-SKYOOL)
From Latin *minusculus,* meaning "smallish."

Also given as **minuscular** (mi-NUS-kyoo-lər), with the same meaning.

1. extremely small.

"How can we condone the tens of millions of dollars spent on this project to achieve **minuscule** gains when the same amount could have been spent on substantial improvements in public housing?"

2. small; not written as capital letters, lowercase.

"My children were encouraged for years to write all their schoolwork in **minuscule** letters and never did achieve comfort in writing ordinary letters, some capitalized, others not."

miscreant (MIS-kree-ənt)
From Middle French *mescreant,* meaning "unbelieving."

depraved, villainous, base.

"The cashier seemed to be such an upstanding citizen that we were shocked to learn of her **miscreant** behavior."

Related words: **miscreance** (MIS-kree-əns) and **miscreancy** (MIS-kree-ən-see) *both nouns.*

mnemonic (ni-MON-ik)
From Greek *mnemonikós,* meaning "relating to memory; mindful."

of or pertaining to memory; intended to aid the memory.

"She was fortunate in mastering certain clever **mnemonic** devices that helped her recall such unimportant facts as the names of all English monarchs in chronological order."

Related words: **mnemonically** (ni-MON-i-kə-lee) *adverb;* **mnemon-**

ics (ni-MON-iks) and **mnemotechnics** (NEE-moh-TEK-niks) *both nouns.*

mollescent (mə-LES-ənt)

From Latin *mollescens,* present participle of *mollescere,* meaning "to soften, become effeminate"; from *mollis,* meaning "soft," + *-escent,* an adjectival suffix.

Revealing for us once again the Romans' perception of women in the male versus female competition.

softening; tending to become soft.

"As he watched, the **mollescent** tissue on his table appeared to evolve into the pulpy state he was waiting to observe."

Related word: **mollescence** (mə-LES-əns).

moonstruck (MOON-STRUK)

From English **moon** + **struck,** past participle of **strike.** One of many mystical allusions to the supposed power of the moon.

Also given as **moonstricken** (MOON-STRIK-ən).

1. hopelessly romantic; lost in the fantasy of love.

"The American musical stage often depicts a pair of **moonstruck** young lovers ensnared by mutual affection and unable to think rationally until the final act."

2. crazed as though by the influence of the moon.

"We watched in dismay as the incongruously **moonstruck** old woman wandered aimlessly in her garden, unaware of her beautiful surroundings."

mordacious (mor-DAY-shəs)

From Latin *mordax,* meaning "biting, sharp"; from infinitive *mordere,* meaning "to bite." *See* **mordant.**

1. biting; given to biting.

"The **mordacious** child, so difficult to control, was refused admission to nursery school."

2. of speech or writing: caustic in style or tone; mordant.

"It is far easier to write **mordacious** book reviews than to write books, a truth that book reviewers seem to forget."

Golden Adjectives

Related words: **mordaciously** (mor-DAY-shəs-lee) *adverb*; **mordacity** (mor-DAS-i-tee) *noun*.

mordant (MOR-dnt)

From Latin infinitive *mordere*, meaning "to bite." *See* **mordacious.**

1. of a speaker or writer: caustic, sarcastic, mordacious.

"Unfortunately, Stanley's conversation was imbued with a **mordant** wit that could not be suppressed even when he tried to be civil."

2. pungent; burning.

"The swimmer's every move seemed to indicate the onset of **mordant** pain, hampering her normally fluid strokes."

Related words: **mordantly** (MOR-dnt-lee) *adverb*; **mordancy** (MOR-dn-see) *noun*.

moribund (MOR-ə-BUND)

From Latin *moribundus*, meaning "dying; mortal; deadly"; from infinitive *mori*, meaning "to die."

1. at the point of death; stagnant, not progressing.

"More than once, **moribund** patients have been revived and, within days, sent home to live through whatever life remained for them."

2. on the verge of extinction.

"The membership had dwindled to the point at which it was no longer feasible to keep the **moribund** institution open."

Related words: **moribundly** (MOR-ə-BUND-lee) *adverb*; **moribundity** (MOR-ə-BUN-di-tee) *noun*.

morose (mə-ROHS)

From Latin *morosus*, meaning "peevish, difficult."

ill-humored: sullen, gloomy; expressing bad humor.

"Bob was so **morose** about the loss of his job that the rest of the family became depressed along with him."

Related words: **morosely** (mə-ROHS-lee) *adverb*; **moroseness** (mə-ROHS-nis) *noun*.

mundane (mun-DAYN)

From Latin *mundanus*, from *mundus*, meaning "clean and neat."

banal; ordinary, common, everyday; earthly: pertaining to this world, not to heaven.

"No matter how distasteful **mundane** responsibilities may seem to the young, such as working for a living or keeping oneself presentable, they give a structure to life that keeps one going."

Related words: **mundanely** (mun-DAYN-lee) *adverb*; **mundaneness** (mun-DAYN-nis) and **mundanity** (mun-DAN-i-tee) *both nouns.*

N

nascent (NAY-sənt)

> From Latin *nascens*, present participle of infinitive *nasci*, meaning "to arise, to be born."

arising; beginning to form; coming into existence.

> "The international agency, recognizing the outpouring of support, did everything possible to encourage the **nascent** democracy."

> Related words: **nascence** (NAY-səns) and **nascency** (NAY-sən-see) *both nouns.*

nauseous (NAW-shəs)

> From Latin *nauseosus* from *nausea*, also given as *nausia*, from Greek *nausía*, meaning "seasickness."

The fastidious—enjoying the game of gotcha—like to cite one or another of the italicized words given in the paragraph above in order to suggest their own correct—actually incorrect—English usage.

It may have started generations ago when an English teacher misled by dreams of lexical eminence saw and grabbed her opportunity for linguistic immortality, proclaiming there was something wrong with **nauseous** that put it beyond the pale. To this day girls and boys passing through the classrooms of ill-advised arbiters of language have been exposed to similar nonsense. Yet, there is nothing wrong with the word **nauseous,** as you will soon see. For hundreds of years, as documented by the editors of the *Oxford English Dictionary*, there has been the word **nauseous,** with its multiple meanings, and always the word of choice for the masses and eschewed by the half educated. Read on.

1. nauseated; sick to one's stomach.

"Within an hour of leaving their home port, all passengers aboard were **nauseous,** to the point of retching, even vomiting."

2. nauseating; sickening, causing nausea.

"The **nauseous** diet they served, particularly the greasy fish and baked insects, killed our appetites."

3. loathsome; disgusting; highly offensive.

"His masterful command of **nauseous** language, which he did not hesitate to employ even in the company of my daughters, did not endear him to me."

Related words: **nauseating** (NAW-zee-AY-ting) *adjective;* **nauseously** (NAW-shəs-lee) *adverb;* **nausea** (NAW-zee-ə) and **nauseousness** (NAW-shəs-nis) *both nouns;* **nauseate** (NAW-zee-AYT) *verb.*

nebulous (NEB-yə-ləs)

From Latin *nebulosis,* meaning "misty, cloudy," from Latin *nebula,* meaning "mist, vapor, cloud."

1. indistinct; vague, hazy, confused; cloudy.

"Because of her relative unfamiliarity with the subjects they had begun to study, Miriam had only a **nebulous** idea of where her efforts might lead."

2. nebular; resembling a cluster of interstellar stars.
"From the time he had first perceived a cloud of **nebulous** material during a session in the observatory, he began to spend all his nights there, trying to identify everything he saw."

Related words: **nebulously** (NEB-yə-ləs-lee) *adverb;* **nebulose** (NEB-yə-lohs) *adjective;* **nebulize** (NEB-yə-LIZ) *verb;* **nebula** (NEB-yə-lə), **nebulousness** (NEB-yə-ləs-nis), and **nebulosity** (NEB-yə-LOS-i-tee) *all nouns.*

necessitous (nə-SES-i-təs)

From the familiar English noun **necessity + -ous,** an adjectival suffix meaning "full of."

impoverished; hard up; poor, needy; requiring assistance, attention, or action.

"We knew from his increasingly **necessitous** demands that his financial situation had worsened since we first had come upon him."

Related words: **necessitously** (nə-SES-i-təs-lee) *adverb*; **necessitate** (nə-SES-i-TAYT) *verb*; **necessity** (nə-SES-i-tee) and **necessitousness** (nə-SES-i-təs-nis) *both nouns.*

nefarious (ni-FAIR-ee-əs)

From Latin *nefarius*, meaning "heinous, criminal"; from *nefas*, meaning "wickedness, sin, wrong"; from *ne-*, a negative prefix, + *fas*, meaning "divine law," + *-ius*, an adjectival suffix.

iniquitous; wicked; villainous.

"They had all conspired for the same **nefarious** purpose, to swindle the charity out of all the proceeds of the bazaar."

Related words: **nefariously** (ni-FAIR-ee-əs-lee) *adverb*; **nefariousness** (ni-FAIR-ee-əs-nis) *noun.*

neoteric (NEE-ə-TER-ik)

From Latin *neotericus*, meaning "new, modern"; from Greek *neoterikós*, meaning "youthful, young."

recent, new; modern.

"Little more can be said for those shameless **neoteric** writers who find no subject too degrading for them to write about."

Related words: **neoterically** (NEE-ə-TER-i-kə-lee) *adverb*; **neoterism** (nee-OT-ə-RIZ-əm) *noun.*

nescient (NESH-ənt)

From Latin *nescientia*, meaning "ignorance"; from *ne-*, meaning "not," + *scientia*, meaning "knowledge."

ignorant; agnostic.

"Only the **nescient** person, whether an ignoramus or an unbeliever, would take no position at all on matters of such importance."

Related word: **nescience** (NESH-əns) *noun.*

nettlesome (NET-l-səm)

From English **nettle,** meaning "a stinging plant," + **-some,** an adjectival suffix.

irritable: easily annoyed.

"In that **nettlesome** teacher's class we had learned to behave warily lest we be punished for some minor infraction."

nice-nelly (NĪS-NEL-ee)

From the given name *Nelly.*

Also given as **nice-Nelly.**

prudish, genteel; excessively prudish or genteel.

"When Stephen realized that Evelyn was always going to be one of those **nice-nelly** girls, he decided he would be better off looking elsewhere."

Related words: **nice-nellyism** or **nice-Nellyism** (NĪS-NEL-ee-IZ-əm) both nouns.

niveous (NIV-ee-əs)

From Latin *niveus,* meaning "snowy; snow-white."

snowy; resembling snow.

"My old cottage looked imposingly dressed, the would-be poet said, just waiting to be escorted to a formal dance in the **niveous** stole of winter."

noctambulous (nok-TAM-byə-ləs)

From Latin *noct-,* a combining form meaning "night," + the infinitive *ambulare,* meaning "to walk, travel," + *-ous.*

Also given as **noctambulant** (nok-TAM-byə-lənt) and as **noctambulistic** (nok-TAM-byə-LIS-tik).

given to sleepwalking.

"We had to make certain that William, who is known to be **noctambulous,** is not assigned an upper berth aboard ship lest he fall to the floor at the start of one of his nightly jaunts."

Related words: **noctambulism** (nok-TAM-byə-LIZ-əm), **noctambulist** (nok-TAM-byə-list), and **noctambule** (nok-TAM-byool) *all nouns.*

nocuous (NOK-yoo-əs)

From Latin *nocuus,* meaning "harmful, injurious," from infinitive *nocere,* meaning "to harm, to hurt" + *-uus* an adjectival suffix.

A tribute to the generosity and competence of our species, in that we hear far more the word **innocuous** than **nocuous.** Could it be because we don't often need to express the latter thought? *See also* **noxious.**

noxious; hurtful; poisonous, venomous.

"She soon became expert at recognizing the differences between edible mushrooms and the many types of **nocuous** ones."

Related words: **nocuously** (NOK-yoo-əs-lee) *adverb;* **nocuousness** (NOK-yoo-əs-nis) *noun.*

noetic (noh-ET-ik)

From Greek *noetikós,* meaning "intelligent," from *nóesis,* meaning "mind," + *-tikos,* an adjectival suffix.

pertaining to the intellect; originating in the mind.

"Jason has not yet reached the stage in intellectual development at which he can express **noetic** perceptions."

Related words: **noesis** (noh-EE-sis) and **noetics** (noh-ET-iks) *both nouns.*

noisome (NOY-səm)

From Middle English *noy,* a form of "annoy," + *-some,* an adjectival suffix.

Notice that **noisome** has nothing to do with "noise," a common misperception.

1. of an odor: ill-smelling; offensive to the sense of smell.

"Generations of illegal dumping have made our once-beautiful New England countrysides the repositories of **noisome** garbage and discarded metals, which pollute our lives and rob us of chances of enjoying health and dignity."

2. harmful; injurious; noxious.

"In ill-lighted, **noisome** cellars all over Chinatown, immigrant women worked for twelve hours a day, seven days a week in order for their children one day to enjoy the benefits of American life."

Related words: **noisomely** (NOY-səm-lee) *adverb;* **noisomeness** (NOY-səm-nis) *noun.*

nonpareil (NON-pə-REL)

From Middle French *nonpareil,* from the prefix *non-,* meaning "not," + *pareil,* meaning "equal."

peerless; having no equal.

"When he actually characterized her unmelodious voice as **nonpareil,** I became aware at once he was either stupid or a charlatan."

noxious (NOK-shəs)

From Latin *noxius,* meaning "harmful, guilty"; from the noun *noxa,* meaning "hurt, damage," + *-ius,* an adjectival suffix. *See also* **nocuous.**

nocuous; injurious, hurtful, harmful; unwholesome.

"Once cool weather sets in, a **noxious** wind can be expected to blow for hours after lunch, so children will have to remain in their classrooms until the wind dies down after dark."

Related words: **noxiously** (NOK-shəs-lee) *adverb;* **noxiousness** (NOK-shəs-nis) *noun.*

nubile (NOO-bīl)

From Latin *nubilis,* meaning "marriageable"; from infinitive *nubere,* meaning "to marry," + *-ilis,* an adjectival suffix expressing capability.

Do not confuse *nubilis,* meaning "marriageable," with *nubilus,* meaning "cloudy" or "gloomy," mentioned in the next entry, no matter how strong the impulse to confuse the two states.

of a young woman: attractive and sexually developed; marriageable.

"You would think the old lady, ever the marriage broker, kept a list of two classifications of candidate girls in her purse, those who were **nubile** and those who were within a year of attaining that state."

Related word: **nubility** (noo-BIL-i-tee) *noun.*

nubilous (NOO-bə-ləs)

From Latin *nubilus,* meaning "cloudy, gloomy"; from the noun *nubes,* meaning "cloud," + *-lus,* an adjectival suffix meaning "full of."

See also **nubile,** which derives from the Latin *nubilis,* meaning "marriageable."

obscure, vague; cloudy, foggy.

"The new manager, not Joe, had only a **nubilous** understanding of what his team was able to accomplish in a short series."

nugacious. *See* nugatory.

nugatory (NOO-gə-TOR-ee)

From Latin *nugatorius,* meaning "futile"; from infinitive *nugari,* meaning "to trifle," + *-torius,* an adjectival suffix.

Also occasionally given as **nugacious** (noo-GAY-shəs), which has the same meanings, but derives from Latin *nugax,* meaning "frivolous."

worthless, useless; futile, vain; not valid.

"Most of the small improvements you are making are **nugatory,** making me think what we need is an overhaul of the entire system."

nuncupative (NUNG-kyə-PAY-tiv)

> From Latin *nuncupatus*, past participle of infinitive *nuncupare*, meaning "to name; declare."

of wills: oral, not written.

> "It long had been the custom to authorize soldiers and sailors on dangerous duty far from their home countries to make **nuncupative** wills, which were considered to be binding and fully within the law."

O

obdurate (OB-duu-rit)

From Latin *obduratus*, past participle of infinitive *obdurare*, meaning "to harden in heart, persist"; from prefix *ob-*, meaning "toward," + *durus*, meaning "hard," + *-atus*, an adjectival suffix. *See also* **indurate**.

unyielding to persuasion; resistant to moral influence; impenitent.

"It all might have gone differently if the son had not been an even more **obdurate** sinner than his father had been."

Related words: **obdurately** (OB-duu-rit-lee) *adverb*; **obdurateness** (OB-duu-rit-nis) and **obduracy** (OB-duu-rue-see) *both nouns*.

objurgatory (ob-JUR-gə-TOR-ee)

From Latin *obiurgatorius*, meaning "reproachful," from infinitive *obiurgare*, meaning "to scold, rebuke."

Also given as **objurgative** (ob-JUR-gə-tiv).

uttering or constituting a scolding or sharp rebuke.

"Her **objurgatory** tone, which she adopted as soon as knew she had been caught, could reduce me to tears."

Related words: **objurgatorily** (ob-JUR-gə-TOR-i-lee) and **objurgatively** (ob-JUR-gə-tiv-lee) *both adverbs*; **objurgation** (OB-jur-GAY-shən) and **objurgator** (OB-jur-GAY-tor) *both nouns*.

oblivious (ə-BLIV-ee-əs)

From Latin *obliviosus*, meaning "forgetful," from infinitive *oblivisci*, meaning "to forget," + *-osus*, an adjectival suffix.

unmindful; unaware or unconscious of; forgetful.

"I voted confidently, convinced my candidate was going to win, and **oblivious** to the hostile, partisan stares I had been exposed to ever since I entered the polling station."

Related words: **obliviously** (ə-BLIV-ee-əs-lee) *adverb*; **oblivion** (ə-BLIV-ee-ən) and **obliviousness** (ə-BLIV-ee-əs-nis) *both nouns*.

obnoxious (əb-NOK-shəs)

From Latin *obnoxiosus*, meaning "submissive"; from *obnoxius*, meaning "exposed to harm."

odious; objectionable; highly offensive.

"The large, noisy party at the next table was **obnoxious** and cast a pall over our evening out."

Related words: **obnoxiously** (əb-NOK-shəs-lee) *adverb*; **obnoxiousness** (əb-NOK-shəs-nis) *noun*.

obsequious (əb-SEE-kwee-əs)

From Latin *obsequiosus*, meaning "compliant, obedient"; from infinitive *obsequi*, meaning "to comply with, yield to."

fawning, showing servility; compliant, deferential, sycophantic; ignobly obedient.

"I was flummoxed by his immediate transformation into an **obsequious** bootlicker when he saw his boss enter the room."

Related words: **obsequiously** (əb-SEE-kwee-əs-lee) *adverb*; **obsequiousness** (əb-SEE-kwee-əs-nis) and **obsequence** (OB-si-kwəns) *both nouns*.

obtrusive (əb-TROO-siv)

From Latin *obtrusus*, past participle of infinitive *obtrudere*, meaning "to force on to."

projecting so as to be in the way; forcing oneself or one's opinions into prominence.

"We agreed we had been astonished to see how **obtrusive** she was in presenting her opinions, obviously thinking such behavior would advance her cause."

Related words: **obtrusively** (əb-TROO-siv-lee) *adverb*; **obtrusiveness** (əb-TROO-siv-nis), **obtrusion** (əb-TROO-zhən), and **obtruder** (əb-TROOD-ər) *all nouns*.

obtuse (əb-TOOS)

From Latin *obtusus*, meaning "dulled," past participle of infinitive *obtundere*, meaning "to beat, to thump."

insensitive; not acutely perceptive.

"Unfortunately, I was entirely too **obtuse** to understand she was trying to express confidence in me by sending me out of the country to open new markets."

Related words: **obtusely** (əb-TOOS-lee) *adverb*; **obtuseness** (əb-TOOS-nis) *noun*.

odious (OH-dee-əs)

From Latin *odiosus*, from *odium*, meaning "hatred, displeasure"; from *odi-* "I hate," + *-osus*, an adjectival suffix meaning "full of."

repulsive; highly offensive; deserving hatred, causing hatred or repugnance.

"The century past was filled paradoxically with some of the most laudable achievements of mankind and some of the most **odious** manifestations of its evil potential."

Related words: **odium** (OH-dee-əm) and **odiousness** (OH-dee-əs-nis) *both nouns*; **odiously** (OH-dee-əs-lee) *adverb*.

oedipal (ED-ə-pəl)

From the name Oedipus, literally meaning "swollen-footed," a legendary Theban hero who unwittingly killed his father, Laius, and married his mother, Jocasta. Neither mother nor son knew of their family relationship.

The adjective **oedipal** would have little to do with the rest of this if Sigmund Freud had not become acquainted with the play *Oedipus Tyrannus*, which Sophocles wrote about the legend.

The plot of the play follows closely the legend of Oedipus and the others, and Freud gave the name **Oedipus complex** to the sexual desire of a son for his mother and, conversely, the hatred of a son for his father, both emotions being unknown to the principals.

Also given as **Oedipal**: characterized by a psychoanalytic complex in which a strong desire is felt for a parent of the opposite sex.

"The powerful final scene of the play clearly identifies the **oedipal** nature of the emotions felt by the protagonist and his mother."

Related words: **Oedipean** (ED-ə-PEE-ən) *adjective;* **Oedipus** (ED-ə-pəs) *noun.*

officious (ə-FISH-əs)

From Latin *officiosus,* meaning "obliging, dutiful." From the Latin *offici(um),* meaning "service, attention," + *-osus,* an adjectival suffix meaning "full of."

Clearly a word that warns us against doing more good than is desired.

meddlesome; offering one's unasked-for help.

"Penny is so **officious** there is no aspect of her sister-in-law's life she does not try to invade and offer to improve through her advice."

Related words: **officiously** (ə-FISH-əs-lee) *adverb;* **officiousness** (ə-FISH-əs-nis) *noun.*

oleaginous (OH-lee-AJ-ə-nəs)

From Latin *oleaginus,* meaning "of the olive tree"; from *olea,* meaning "olive tree."

Oil has made wheels turn smoothly and salads taste better in societies from pre-Roman times to the present, possibly into the foreseeable future. So why can one oily olive differ from other oily olives? Simple, too much oil. And in this case when oil becomes too much oil, it becomes a hindrance—fatty, greasy—instead of a help. Hence the most important meaning of **oleaginous.**

unctuous; fawning; fatty, greasy.

"My mother wanted to be ingratiating, but her **oleaginous** manner was truly repellent."

Related word: **oleaginousness** (OH-lee-AJ-ə-nəs-nis) *noun.*

olfactory (ol-FAK-tə-ree)

From Latin *olfactorius,* from the infinitive *olfacere,* meaning "to smell at"; from *olere,* meaning "to smell," + *facere,* meaning "to make," + *-torius,* an adjectival suffix.

pertaining to the sense of smell.

"The laboratory where Elaine works is concerned solely with **olfactory** experiments, mostly leading to selection of various contemplated scents."

Related words: **olfactorily** (ol-FAK-tə-ri-lee) *adverb;* **olfaction** (ol-FAK-shən) *noun.*

ominous (OM-ə-nəs)

> From Latin *ominosus*, meaning "portentous"; from *omen*, meaning "omen," + *-osus*, an adjectival suffix meaning "possessing."

inauspicious; foreboding evil.

> "Shortly before the beginning of the championship game we were given the **ominous** news that several of our players had failed their drug tests and would be kept off the team."

> Related words: **ominously** (OM-i-nəs-lee) *adverb*; **ominousness** (OM-ə-nə-nis) *noun*.

onerous (ON-ər-əs)

> From Latin *onerosus*, meaning "heavy, burdensome, irksome"; from *onus*, meaning "load, burden," + *-osus*, an adjectival suffix meaning "full of."

burdensome; oppressive, troublesome; of the nature of a legal obligation.

> "The duties of the U.S. president are so **onerous** that one must wonder why so many people seem to aspire to that office."

> Related words: **onerously** (ON-ər-əs-lee) adverb; **onerousness** (ON-ər-əs-nis) *noun*.

opalescent (OH-pə-LES-ənt)

> From English **opal,** meaning "a type of gem," + **-escent**, an adjectival suffix.

iridescent; exhibiting a play of colors of an opal; having a milky play of changing colors.

> "The sea and sky along with softly colored buildings combine to give Venice an **opalescent** glow."

> Related words: **opalesce** (OH-pə-LES) *verb*; **opalescently** (OH-pə-LES-ənt-lee) *adverb*; **opalescence** (OH-pə-LES-əns) *noun*.

operose (OP-ə-ROHS)

> From Latin *operosus*, meaning "industrious, active; laborious, elaborate"; from *opus*, meaning "a work; workmanship; building."

of a person: industrious; of a task: tedious; done with much labor.

> "It did not take them long to devise a plan that was much less **operose** and could be done quickly."

> Related words: **operosely** (OP-ə-ROHS-lee) *adverb*; **operoseness** (OP-ə-ROHS-nis) *noun*.

opiate (OH-pee-it)

From Medieval Latin *opiatus,* meaning "bringing sleep," past participle of infinitive *opiare,* meaning "to cause sleep."

Opiate is often used as a noun.

soporific; narcotic, inducing sleep; inducing drowsiness.

"A splendid lecture delivered inaudibly in a monotone and covering a subject certain to be excluded from the final examination has an **opiate** effect on most classes."

Related word: **opiatic** (OH-pee-AT-ik) *adjective.*

oppidan (OP-i-dən)

From Latin *oppidanus,* meaning "provincial"; from *oppidum,* meaning "town."

Also used as a noun: "He was known as an **oppidan.**"

urban; of a town, as opposed to the country.

"Try as he would, he was unable to make people think he was an **oppidan** type rather than the hick he thought he had outgrown."

opprobrious (ə-PROH-bree-əs)

From Late Latin *opprobriosus,* from Latin *opprobrium,* a noun meaning "disgrace, reproach, scandal"; from *opprobare,* meaning "to taunt."

contumelious; vituperative; conveying injurious reproach.

"The speaker was subjected to **opprobrious** cries that subsided only when he completely stopped speaking and sat down, a chastened man."

Related words: **opprobriously** (ə-PROH-bree-əs-lee) *adverb;* **opprobrium** (ə-PROH-bree-əm) and **opprobriousness** (ə-PROH-bree-əs-nis) *both nouns.*

oppugnant (ə-PUG-nənt)

From Latin *oppugnans,* present participle of *oppugnare,* meaning "to attack, to assault."

opposing, antagonistic, contrary, repugnant.

"Suggestions that we consider splitting the marketing department in three were immediately derided as **oppugnant** to the individual interests of all members of the group."

Related word: **oppugnancy** (ə-PUG-nən-see) *noun.*

oracular (aw-RAK-yə-lər)
From Latin *oraculum,* meaning "oracle, prophecy."

1. of a person: speaking or writing as though he or she were an oracle.

"I am tired of the opinions and predictions delivered by the so-called **oracular** pundits, who actually know little more than you and I."

2. of a statement: sententious; delivered as though by divine inspiration; ominous, infallible.

"After a while we realized that his **oracular** opinions were based on nothing more than his hunches and personal prejudices."

3. ambiguous, obscure.

"His sports predictions were made intentionally **oracular** to enable him to claim second sight no matter which side won."

Related words: **oracularly** (aw-RAK-yə-lər-lee) *adverb*; **oracle** (OR-ə-kəl), **oracularity** (aw-RAK-yə-LAR-i-tee), and **oracularness** (aw-RAK-yə-lər-nis) *all nouns.*

ordurous (OR-jə-rəs)
From Middle English and Middle French *ord,* meaning "filthy"; from Latin *horridus,* meaning "horrid."

of the nature of excrement or dung; filthy.

"Little boys Jonny's age took great delight in displaying their **ordurous** vocabularies."

Related word: **ordure** (OR-jər) *noun.*

orotund (OR-ə-TUND)
From Latin phrase *ore rotundo,* literally translated as "with round mouth"; meaning "with round, well-turned speech."

1. of the voice or speech: full, rich, strong.

"As soon as James began to sing, it was obvious that his classical training had given him a resonant, **orotund** voice."

2. of speaking style: magniloquent; inflated or pompous; bombastic.

"Instead of being treated to a talk rich in meaning we were confronted by an **orotund** linguistic display devoid of good sense."

Related word: **orotundity** (OR-ə-TUN-di-tee) *noun.*

oscitant (OS-i-tənt)

From Latin *oscitans*, present participle of *oscitare*, meaning "to be drowsy, yawn."

gaping from drowsiness, yawning; drowsy, dull, indolent, inattentive, negligent.

"From their **oscitant** demeanor, I wondered whether they were bored or possibly drugged."

Related words: **oscitancy** (OS-i-tən-see) and **oscitance** (OS-i-təns) *both nouns.*

ostensible (o-STEN-sə-bəl)

From Latin *ostensus* or *ostentus*, past participle of infinitive *ostendere*, meaning "to hold out, display, reveal."

Also given as **ostensive** (o-STEN-siv).

professed, pretended; intended, evident.

"His **ostensible** purpose was to interview the rebel leader for the press, masking his intention to assassinate the man."

Related words: **ostensibly** (o-STEN-sə-blee) and **ostensively** (o-STEN-siv-lee) *both adverbs.*

ostentatious (os-ten-TAY-shəs)

From English **ostentation**; from Latin *ostentatio*, from *ostentatus*, past participle of infinitive *ostendere*, meaning "to hold out, display, reveal." *See also* **ostensible.**

of manners, etc.: calculated to attract notice; of a person: given to conspicuous show.

"The new widower had established himself next to the open casket in an attitude of **ostentatious** bereavement, with an intensity that rose each time an attractive young woman drew near."

Related words: **ostentatiously** (os-ten-TAY-shəs-lee) *adverb;* **ostentation** (os-ten-TAY-shən) and **ostentatiousness** (os-ten-TAY-shəs-nis) *both nouns.*

otiose (OH-shee-ohs)

From Latin *otiosus*, meaning "at leisure, unemployed; out of public affairs."

1. indolent; lazy; unemployed, idle.

"Many of the men and women seen smoking behind the student center are not students at all, but **otiose** dropouts with nothing better to do."

2. nugatory; superfluous, futile, ineffective.

"You are wrong to think an action of the kind I have been discussing is completely **otiose,** rather than helpful to our cause."

outré (oo-TRAY)

From French past participle of *outrer,* meaning "to go beyond limits; push to excess."

unconventional, bizarre, unusual, eccentric; beyond what is considered correct.

"Although some of Emily's critics found her work **outré,** most thought it original and worthy of consideration."

overriding (OH-vər-RĪ-ding)

From English **over** + **ride,** meaning "to prevail."

dominating; taking precedence over other considerations.

"My **overriding** concern is that harm not befall the innocent children no matter what provocation they give you."

oversolicitous (OH-vər-sə-LIS-i-təs)

From English **over** + **solicitous,** meaning "concerned."

excessively or unduly solicitous.

"The actions of **oversolicitous** parents can cause even more damage than that caused by parents who show insufficient concern."

overweening (OH-vər-WEE-ning)

From Middle English *overwening,* from *ofer,* meaning "over," + *wenen,* meaning "to expect."

excessively conceited; overconfident or proud; arrogant; excessive, exaggerated.

"I always wondered how one so young could exhibit such **overweening** self-confidence even though his record was well below average."

Related words: **overweeningly** (OH-vər-WEE-ning-lee) *adverb;* **overweeningness** (OH-vər-WEE-ning-nis) *noun.*

overwrought (OH-vər-RAWT)

From Middle English *ofer,* meaning "over," + *wroght,* past participle of *worchen,* meaning "to work."

1. excessively excited or agitated.

"My aunt would not let Grandma watch wrestling on television because she thought it left the old lady **overwrought**."

2. excessively ornate.

"When I realized my writing had become **overwrought**, I set about trying to simplify my style."

P

pachydermatous (PAK-i-DUR-mə-təs)

From Greek *pachy*, meaning "thick," + *-dermatos*, a suffix meaning "skinned."

1. thick-skinned; insensitive to rebuff or to external abuses.

"A person as **pachydermatous** as he cannot be expected to understand that his attentions are not welcome."

2. characteristic of an elephant and other creatures like it.

"The huge, lumbering **pachydermatous** creature showed remarkable ability to locate and follow its small prey."

Related word: **pachydermatously** (PAK-i-DUR-mə-təs-lee) *adverb;* **pachyderm** (PAK-i-DURM) *noun;* **pachydermal** (PAK-i-DUR-məl), **pachydermous** (PAK-i-DUR-məs), and **pachydermic** (PAK-i-DUR-mik) *all adjectives.*

palliative (PAL-ee-ə-tiv)

From French *palliatif*, meaning "palliative"; from Latin *palliativus*, past participle of infinitive *palliare*, meaning "to cloak, cover."

ameliorative; serving to relieve (disease, etc.) temporarily.

"Until discovery of antibiotics, drugs were considered merely **palliative** rather than curative, at best controlling excessive body temperature."

Related words: **palliatively** (PAL-ee-ə-tiv-lee) *adverb;* **palliate** (PAL-ee-AYT) *verb;* **palliation** (PAL-ee-AY-shən) and **palliator** (PAL-ee-AY-tər) *both nouns.*

pallid (PAL-id)

From Latin *pallidus*, meaning "pale, sallow," from infinitive *pallere*, meaning "to be pale," + *-idus*, an adjectival suffix.

1. unspirited; lacking liveliness.

"Technical competence will not be sufficient to outweigh his **pallid** interpretation of great music."

2. wan; deficient in color.

"Her **pallid** complexion was an uncharacteristic sign of possible physical problems that would have to be investigated."

Related words: **pallidly** (PAL-id-lee) *adverb*; **pallidness** (PAL-id-nis) *noun*.

palpable (PAL-pǝ-bǝl)

From Latin *palpabilis*, meaning "which can be touched"; from infinitive *palpare*, meaning "to caress, coax, flatter."

1. tangible; sensible; capable of being touched or felt.

"A competent physician employing no more than her sense of touch can often detect **palpable** conditions indicating the presence of certain physical abnormalities."

2. noticeable; readily perceptible.

"The average juror may think that a shifty-eyed witness is a **palpable** perjurer and should not be trusted.

Do not confuse **palpable** with **palpebral** (see below).

Related words: **palpably** (PAL-pǝ-blee) *adverb*; **palpability** (PAL-pǝ-BIL-i-tee) and **palpableness** (PAL-pǝ-bǝl-nis) *both nouns.*

palpebral (PAL-pǝ-brǝl)

From Latin *palpebralis*, meaning "of the eyelids," from *palpebra*, meaning "eyelid." Do not confuse with **palpable.**

pertaining to the eyelids.

"His rapid **palpebral** fluttering occurred most often when he was deep in thought and close to a decision."

Related word: **palpebrate** (PAL-pǝ-BRAYT) *adjective.*

palsied (PAWL-zeed)

From English **palsy,** meaning "a form of paralysis."

paralyzed; afflicted by palsy; unable to control certain muscles.

"His **palsied** movements made many relatively simple tasks difficult for him."

Related word: **palsy** (PAWL-zee) *noun.*

paludal (pə-LOOD-l)

From Latin *palus*, meaning "swamp, marsh, lake."

pertaining to a marsh; arising from or produced by a marsh.

"The heroine of the novel had been warned she could expect to encounter malaria if she insisted on spending summers so close to Rome, but she ignored the warning and soon contracted the **paludal** disease."

pandemic (pan-DEM-ik)

From Latin *pandemus*, from Greek *pándemos*, meaning "public, common"; from *pan-*, meaning "all," + *demos*, meaning "the people," + *-os*, an adjectival suffix.

There is general confusion over the meaning of the word **epidemic** (EP-i-DEM-ik) and near-total ignorance of the word **pandemic**. Learn first that a **pandemic** (noun) or a **pandemic** (adjective) disease is extremely widespread. Learn also that an **epidemic** (noun) or **epidemic** (adjective) disease is confined, although it may be part of a worldwide **pandemic** (noun). So **epidemic** connotes limitation to a smaller area than **pandemic**.

1. of a disease: encountered throughout a country, continent, or the entire world.

"My father talked often about the epidemic flu—he meant **pandemic** flu—that he lived through in 1918, when more than 20 million people died."

2. universal, general; epidemic over a wide area.

"In the twentieth century we were treated to journalistic invention of a **pandemic** condition called Beatlemania, which was characterized by screaming, sometimes fainting young women."

Related word: **pandemicity** (PAN-də-MIS-i-tee) *noun.*

panegyrical (PAN-i-JIR-i-kəl)

From Latin *panegyricus*, meaning "of a public eulogy," from Greek *panegyrikós*, meaning "fit for a public festival"; from *panégyris*, meaning "solemn assembly."

eulogistic; encomiastic, laudatory; publicly or elaborately expressing praise.

"The **panegyrical** funeral oration was entirely fitting for a person who had made a truly great contribution to modern life."

Related words: **panegyrically** (PAN-i-JIR-i-kə-lee) *adverb*; **panegyric** (PAN-i-JIR-ik) and **panegyrist** (PAN-i-JIR-ist) *both nouns*; **panegyrize** (PAN-i-jə-RĪz) *verb*.

See also **encomiastic.**

Panglossian (pan-GLOS-ee-ən)

From *Pangloss*, the name of the naive tutor-philosopher in Voltaire's eighteenth-century novel *Candide*, who coined the impossibly optimistic legend "All is for the best in this best of all possible worlds." The name Pangloss is from Greek *panglossia*, meaning "wordiness."

unduly optimistic, especially when facing overwhelming odds.

"Will, who knew what life held for an unemployed person of middle age, was exasperated by his mother's **Panglossian** outlook on life."

Paphian (PAY-fee-ən)

From Latin *Paphius*, from Greek *Páphios*, variously meaning "of Paphos, of Aphrodite (Roman) or of Venus (Greek)." Paphos was a city of Cyprus, where the goddess Aphrodite was worshiped.

The lowercase English noun **paphian** means "a prostitute"; we also recall that the words "aphrodisiac" and "anaphrodisiac" are linguistically related to "Aphrodite."

erotic; devoted to unlawful sexual love; pertaining to Aphrodite or to the worship of Aphrodite.

"Countless stories were told of Oscar's campus apartment, where **Paphian** orgies were said to be the rule of the day and the night and made college life palatable during the long, desolate winter."

parietal (pə-RĪ-ə-tl)

From Latin *parietalis*, meaning "of or belonging to walls."

Beyond several biological and anatomical meanings, there is a single meaning of this term that is known or ought to be known by every undergraduate who goes to college away from home and its inevitable restrictions.

having authority over visitation regulations within the walls of a college or university campus.

"In the past decade, **parietal** regulations at our most distinguished undergraduate institutions have been relaxed to a great degree, and the general public has no idea of whether such relaxation has improved or harmed student life."

parsimonious (PAHR-sə-MOH-nee-əs)

From English **parsimony,** meaning "stinginess."

frugal; stingy, avaricious; careful in the use of money.

"How surprised Edna was when her new husband showed his true colors—he was **parsimonious** to a fault, completely uncharitable, and seemingly possessed by the need to invest every penny he could put his hands on."

Related words: **parsimony** (PAHR-sə-MOH-nee) and **parsimoniousness** (PAHR-sə-MOH-nee-əs-nis) *both nouns;* **parsimoniously** (PAHR-sə-MOH-nee-əs-lee) *adverb.*

partible (PAHR-tə-bəl)

From Latin *partibilis,* meaning "divisible," from infinitive *partiri,* meaning "to divide."

separable, divisible: capable of being separated or parted.

"The law made it certain their father's land would be **partible** even though partition in the manner required would surely rob the estate of much of its value to the heirs."

Related word: **partibility** (PAHR-tə-BIL-i-tee) *noun.*

parturient (pahr-TUUR-ee-ənt)

From Latin *parturiens,* meaning "being in labor," present participle of infinitive *parturire,* meaning "to be in labor, to be pregnant."

1. bearing fruit; about to bring forth a child or to give birth.

"It did not take long for the physician to realize that her young patient was **parturient** and in immediate need of attention by a well-prepared team of doctors and nurses."

2. ready to bring forth or produce an idea, etc.

"Once a week the staff of ten **parturient** writers got together for one hour to select the theme for the next broadcast."

Related words: **parturiency** (pahr-TUUR-ee-ən-see) and **parturition** (PAHR-tuu-RISH-ən) *both nouns.*

patulous (PACH-ə-ləs)

From Latin *patulus,* meaning "spreading, broad; standing wide open"; from infinitive *patere,* meaning "to be open, extend."

said often of the boughs of a tree: open, expanded, rather widely open.

"His **patulous** lips, unusually large and always in motion, produced flurries of words that said much and meant little."

Related words: **patulously** (PACH-ə-ləs-lee) *adverb*; **patulousness** (PACH-ə-ləs-nis) *noun*.

pavid (PAV-id)

From Latin *pavidus*, meaning "quaking, terrified," from infinitive *pavere*, meaning "to quake with fear; to dread."

afraid, fearful, frightened.

"The kindergarten teacher had no idea the children would be so **pavid** in the Halloween horrors house that they could not control their screams and shrieks."

Related word: **pavidity** (pə-VID-i-tee) *noun*.

pavonine (PAV-ə-NĪN)

From Latin *pavoninus*, from *pavo*, meaning "peacock."

of, like, or resembling a peacock or its colors.

"He enjoyed watching the old ladies make their entrances through the ballroom doors, parading like **pavonine** latter-day saints."

peccable (PEK-ə-bəl)

From Medieval Latin *peccabilis*, from infinitive *peccare*, meaning "to sin, go wrong."

The infinitive form, given here, is the progenitor of the famous *Peccavi*, "I have sinned," a single word in Latin, three in English, signaling that the declaimer is about to spill the beans. In the unlikely event there is nothing to show or tell, we speak of that person's moral record as being **impeccable.**

capable of sinning, liable to sin.

"Let him who has never been **peccable** cast the first pellet."

Related word: **peccability** (PEK-ə-BIL-i-tee) *noun*.

See also **peccant**.

peccant (PEK-ənt)

From Latin *peccans*, present participle of infinitive *peccare*, meaning "to sin, go wrong."

sinning; offending; faulty, wrong; violating a rule.

"When confronted by clear evidence of **peccant** behavior, the two scoundrels fell to their knees almost simultaneously, each pointing at the other and saying, 'He told me to do it.'"

Related words: **peccantly** (PEK-ənt-lee) *adverb*; **peccancy** (PEK-ən-see) and **peccantness** (PEK-ənt-nis) *both nouns*.

Pecksniffian (pek-SNIF-ee-ən)

From fictional name Seth *Pecksniff*, a character in Dickens's nineteenth-century novel *Martin Chuzzlewit*.

Dickens characterized Pecksniff as a "paltry, despicable" person. Also given as **Pecksniffish** (PEK-snif-ish).

unctuously hypocritical and habitually boasting of benevolence, etc.

"Our congregation had its fill of one **Pecksniffian** loudmouth, who boasted of his charitable nature because, like a Rockefeller, he habitually gave dimes to pathetic vagrants."

Related words: **Pecksniffism** (PEK-snif-iz-əm) and **Pecksniffianism** (pek-SNIF-ee-ən-iz-əm) *both nouns*.

pedicular (pə-DIK-yə-lər)

From Latin *pedicularis* from *pediculus*, diminutive of *pedis*, meaning "a louse," + -*cule* a diminutive adjectival suffix.

Also given as **pediculous** (pə-DIK-yə-ləs).

lousy; of or pertaining to lice.

"Once a **pedicular** outbreak was reported, the school nurse began to make a systematic inspection of the condition of our children's scalps."

Related words: **pediculicide** (pə-DIK-yə-lə-SĪD) *adjective and noun*; **pediculosis** (pə-DIK-yə-LOH-sis) *noun*.

pedophiliac (PEE-də-FIL-ee-ak)

From English **pedophilia**, meaning "pertaining to an abnormal sexual desire in an adult for a child."

Also given as **pedophilic** (PEE-də-FIL-ik).

of, pertaining to, or given to an abnormal sexual desire in an adult for a child.

"Rumors of a **pedophiliac** vagrant in the neighborhood caused near-panic among the parents."

Related words: **pedophilia** (PEE-də-FIL-ee-ə) and **pedophile** (PEE-də-FĪL) *both nouns.*

pejorative (pi-JOR-ə-tiv)

From Latin *peioratus*, past participle of infinitive *peiorare*, meaning "to worsen," from *peior*, meaning "worse."

disparaging; having a derogatory or belittling effect.

"Our dean never missed an opportunity to say something **pejorative** about any candidate for promotion whom he had not himself nominated."

Related words: **pejoratively** (pi-JOR-ə-tiv-lee) *adverb;* **pejoration** (PEJ-ə-RAY-shən) *noun.*

pelagic (pə-LAJ-ik)

From Latin *pelagicus*, from Greek *pelagikós*, meaning "of the open sea"; from *pelag*, "the sea," + *-ikos*, an adjectival suffix.

oceanic; living on or near the surface of the sea.

"The richness of **pelagic** life seemed always to excite experienced divers and the crew members who tended their mother boats."

pellucid (pə-LOO-sid)

From Latin *pellucidus*, a variant form of *perlucidus*, meaning "transparent, bright"; from infinitive *perlucere*, meaning "to shine through."

1. limpid, clear in writing style, in expression.

"Her seemingly effortless, **pellucid** style was actually the product of much painstaking work."

2. translucent, transparent; like glass, allowing maximum passage of light.

"Imagine his delight when he realized the sea was **pellucid** beneath the surface, enabling him to see great schools of delightfully colored fish."

Related words: **pellucidly** (pə-LOO-sid-lee) *adverb;* **pellucidity** (PEL-oo-SID-i-tee) and **pellucidness** (pə-LOO-sid-nis) *both nouns.*

pendulous (PEN-jə-ləs)

From Latin *pendulus*, meaning "hanging, swinging"; from Latin infinitive *pendere*, meaning "to hang, depend, be suspended," + **-ulous,** an adjectival English suffix meaning "habitually engaging in."

1. hanging down loosely; swinging freely, oscillating.

"Since these birds' nests are always suspended from above, they will always be **pendulous** and one day will probably fall."

2. wavering; vacillating, undecided.

"As long as you appear to be **pendulous** whenever a vote is scheduled, you cannot hope to acquire leadership in our legislature."

Related words: **pendulously** (PEN-jə-ləs-lee) *adverb*; **pendulousness** (PEN-jə-ləs-nis) and **pendulum** (PEN-jə-ləm) *both nouns*.

penultimate (pi-NUL-tə-mit)

From Latin *paene*, meaning "almost," + *ultima* or *ultimus*, meaning "last."

next before the last of a series.

"I was surprised to realize I had reached the **penultimate** chapter of her latest book and until that point had found nothing suggesting there would be a logical resolution of the plot."

Related word: **penult** (PEE-nult) *noun*.

penurious (pə-NUUR-ee-əs)

From Latin *penuria*, meaning "a want, a need."

1. parsimonious; stingy; miserly.

"His **penurious** mode of living may have gratified some instinct within him, but the rest of us found his miserly behavior difficult to understand."

2. indigent; destitute, extremely poverty-stricken.

"Despite everything he had done to conserve his small inheritance, by the time he reached old age he was **penurious**, lacking even enough to pay his rent and buy the loaves of bread he lived on."

Related words: **penuriously** (pə-NUUR-ee-əs-lee) *adverb*; **penuriousness** (pə-NUUR-ee-əs-nis) *noun*.

percipient (pər-SIP-ee-ənt)

From Latin *percipiens*, present participle of infinitive *percipere*, meaning "to perceive, get hold of, learn."

discerning; discriminating; capable of grasping; conscious.

"I never fail to marvel at **percipient** critics whose sensitive minds are instantly alert to the insights of the novelists they study."

Related words: **percipience** (pər-SIP-ee-əns) and **percipiency** (pər-SIP-ee-ən-see) *both nouns*.

perdurable (pər-DUUR-ə-bəl)

From Late Latin *perdurabilis*, from infinitive *perdurare*, meaning "to endure, hold out"; from infinitive *durare*, meaning "to stiffen; make hardy."

imperishable; very durable; permanent; eternal, everlasting.

"The ancient Romans looked upon themselves as **perdurable** and could not conceive of a time when the Roman Empire would no longer exist."

Related words: **perdure** (pər-DUUR) *verb*; **perdurably** (pər-DUUR-ə-blee) *adverb*; **perdurability** (pər-DUUR-ə-BIL-i-tee) and **perdurableness** (pər-DUUR-ə-bəl-nis) *both nouns.*

peregrine (PER-i-grin)

From Latin *peregrinus*, meaning "foreign, strange"; from the adverb *peregre*, meaning "abroad, away from home"; from *per-*, a prefix meaning "through," + *ager*, a noun meaning "field, territory."

foreign, alien; belonging to another country; strange, outlandish.

"The native wildflowers in our meadow are being strangled by **peregrine** plants introduced by well-meaning neighbors."

Related words: **peregrinate** (PER-i-grə-NAYT) *verb*; **peregrinator** (PER-i-grə-NAY-tər) and **peregrinity** (PER-i-GRIN-i-tee) *both nouns.*

peremptory (pə-REMP-tə-ree)

From Latin *peremptorius*, meaning "deadly, mortal, destructive"; from *peremptus*, past participle of infinitive *perimere*, meaning "to kill, destroy, prevent."

1. incontrovertible; settling the matter.

"The **peremptory** judgment of the court appeared to deliver a definitive answer to the town's biggest problem."

2. obstinate; stubborn; self-willed.

"When you insist on being **peremptory**, it is impossible to arrive at an amicable agreement."

3. dogmatic: overconfident; intolerant of contradiction.

"Again and again Herbert adopted the **peremptory** attitude that repelled many of those attending the meeting."

Related words: **peremptorily** (pə-REMP-tə-rə-lee) *adverb*; **peremptoriness** (pə-REMP-tə-ree-nis) *noun.*

perfervid (pər-FUR-vid)

From Modern Latin *perfervidus*, from *fervidus*, meaning "hot; fiery; violent," + *per-*, meaning "very."

impassioned; very fervent; glowing, ardent.

"She found the time to pursue her **perfervid** interest in art by never missing a chance to spend her weekends in museums and art galleries."

Related words: **perfervidly** (pər-FUR-fid-lee) *adverb*; **perfervidity** (pər-fər-VID-i-tee), **perfervidness** (pər-FUR-vid-nis), and **perfervor** (pər-FUR-vər) *all nouns.*

perfunctory (pər-FUNGK-tə-ree)

From Late Latin *perfunctorius*, from infinitive *perfungi*, meaning "to perform, discharge, get done with."

1. apathetic; lacking interest, care, or enthusiasm.

"Selma and I thought we were shown only the smallest of courtesies when we received a **perfunctory** thank-you after I returned the lost wallet."

2. hasty and superficial; performed merely as a routine duty.

"I needed less than a few minutes to read his **perfunctory** evaluation of the paper I had worked over for so many hours."

Related words: **perfunctorily** (pər-FUNGK-tə-rə-lee) *adverb*; **perfunctoriness** (pər-FUNGK-tə-ree-nis) *noun.*

peripatetic (PER-ə-pə-TET-ik)

From Latin *peripateticus*, from Greek *peripatetikós*, literally meaning "walking about," and translated as "given to walking about."

An allusion to the habit of Aristotle, a man given to walking about while teaching his students in the Lyceum of Athens.

itinerant; walking or traveling about as, for example, a peddler going from door to door.

"Many of the successful department stores in the New World had their start in the **peripatetic** efforts of determined hawkers of clothing, pots and pans, and the like."

Related word: **peripatetically** (PER-ə-pə-TET-i-kə-lee) *adverb.*

pernicious (pər-NISH-əs)

From Latin *perniciosus*, meaning "ruinous"; from *pernicies*, meaning "destruction, ruin, death."

1. ruinous; causing treacherous harm; hurtful.

"After years of hiding behind a facade of wealth and respectability, Susan was exposed as a **pernicious** schemer."

2. fatal; deadly.

"Physicians attending the old poet began to see signs of anemia and soon identified his illness as **pernicious** anemia, a condition they could not treat at that time."

Related words: **perniciously** (pər-NISH-əs-lee) *adverb*; **perniciousness** (pər-NISH-əs-nis) *noun*.

perspicacious (PUR-spi-KAY-shəs)
From English **perspicacity**, meaning "discernment, penetration"; from Latin infinitive *perspicere*, meaning "to look through, look closely into." *See also* **perspicuous**.

discerning; having keen mental perception; clear-sighted.

"Ellen was thought by her colleagues to be an outstanding person of **perspicacious** judgment."

Related words: **perspicaciously** (PUR-spi-KAY-shəs-lee) *adverb*; **perspicacity** (PUR-spi-KAS-i-tee) and **perspicaciousness** (PUR-spi-KAY-shəs-nis) *both nouns*.

perspicuous (pər-SPIK-yoo-əs)
From Latin *perspicuus*, meaning "transparent; clear, evident"; from infinitive *perspicere*, meaning "to look through, look closely into." *See also* **perspicacious**.

lucid; easy to understand; evident; perspicacious.

"Even a beginning law student could usually grasp the **perspicuous** opinions written by Justice Stevens."

Related words: **perspicuously** (pər-SPIK-yoo-əs-lee) *adverb*; **perspicuity** (PUR-spi-KYOO-i-tee) and **perspicuousness** (pər-SPIK-yoo-əs-nis) *both nouns*.

pertinacious (PUR-tn-AY-shəs)
From English **pertinacity**, from Latin *pertinacia*, meaning "perseverance, stubbornness"; from Latin *pertinax*, meaning "unyielding, stubborn."

1. resolute; holding to a position determinedly.

"The admirably **pertinacious** manner of the young politician alerted us to the likelihood that one day she would hold an important office."

2. obstinate; objectionably persistent.

"His **pertinacious** way of pursuing the meaning of every jot of evidence, no matter how minuscule, drives judges up the wall."

Related words: **pertinaciously** (PUR-tn-AY-shəs-lee) *adverb*; **pertinacity** (PUR-tn-AS-i-tee) and **pertinaciousness** (PUR-tn-AY-shəs-nis) *both nouns.*

perverse (pər-VURS)

From Latin *perversus*, meaning "awry; wrong, perverse"; past participle of infinitive *pervertere*, meaning "to overthrow, overturn, upset."

contrary, obstinate, cantankerous; disposed to go counter to what is expected or espoused.

"Jerome Daly has become so **perverse** that he challenges everything proposed at our board meetings."

Related words: **perversely** (pər-VURS-lee) *adverb*; **perverseness** (pər-VURS-nis) and **perversity** (pər-VUR-si-tee) *both nouns.*

pervicacious (PUR-vi-KAY-shəs)

From Latin *pervicax*, meaning "dogged, stubborn, willful"; from infinitive *pervincere*, meaning "to conquer."

refractory; obstinate; extremely willful; stubborn.

"A truly **pervicacious** opponent in debate, you will find, never gives in under any conditions."

Related words: **pervicaciously** (PUR-vi-KAY-shəs-lee) *adverb*; **pervicaciousness** (PUR-vi-KAY-shəs-nis) *noun.*

pervious (PUR-vee-əs)

From Latin *pervius*, meaning "passable, accessible."

This is one of those adjectives that are far better known in the negative, **impervious** (im-PUR-vee-əs), than in the positive sense, as here. But in the second sense below, see how it opens discussion to a sense that must not be ignored.

1. permeable; allowing of passage through it.

"Fortunately, the selected cloth shielded seedlings from the hot sun but still was **pervious** to rain."

2. intelligible; open to reason or argument.

"George apparently thought that nobody in the entire world but the speaker himself was fully **pervious** to new attitudes or hypotheses."

Related word: **perviousness** (PUR-vee-əs-nis) *noun.*

pettifogging (PET-ee-FOG-ing)

From English **pettifog**, meaning "bicker, quibble"; from Middle Dutch *pettifogger*, meaning "a fixer, one who arranges things."

petty; insignificant, shifty; unethical even in minor matters.

"A miscreant I cannot abide is the **pettifogging** thief who openly shoplifts candy and robs poor boxes yet never admits to committing armed robbery."

Related words: **pettifog** (PET-ee-fog) *verb;* **pettifogger** (PET-ee-FOG-ər) and **pettifoggery** (PET-ee-FOG-ə-ree) *both nouns.*

petulant (PECH-ə-lənt)

From Latin *petulans,* meaning "pert, impudent; lascivious."

displaying peevish impatience.

"She's the kind of person who takes an hour to choose a pair of shoes she wants and then is surprised to find her salesperson is somewhat **petulant**."

Related words: **petulance** (PECH-ə-ləns) and **petulancy** (PECH-ə-lən-see) *both nouns;* **petulantly** (PECH-ə-lənt-lee) *adverb.*

phlegmatic (fleg-MAT-ik)

From Late Latin *phlegmaticus,* from Greek *phlegmatikós,* meaning "pertaining to phlegm," phlegm being a bodily humor thought when excessive to induce apathy.

Also given as **phlegmatical** (fleg-MAT-i-kəl).

sluggish, apathetic; lacking enthusiasm; cool, collected.

"It seemed as if David was born **phlegmatic,** since from his earliest days he never showed interest or excitement for anything that intrigues ordinary mortals."

Related words: **phlegm** (flem) *noun;* **phlegmatically** (fleg-MAT-i-kə-lee) *adverb;* **phlegmaticalness** (fleg-MAT-i-kəl-nis) and **phlegmaticness** (fleg-MAT-ik-nis) *both nouns.*

phocine (FOH-sin)

From Latin *phoca,* from Greek *phóke,* both meaning the animal known as "a seal."

seallike, of or pertaining to seals.

"The primary **phocine** area at our local zoo attracts crowds whenever the weather is good, accommodating adults as well as children who are fascinated by marvelous displays of diving and underwater swimming."

Related word: **phocomelia** (FOH-koh-MEE-lee-ə) *noun.*

phrenetic. *See* **frenetic.**

piacular (pī-AK-yə-lər)
>   From Latin *piacularis*, an adjective meaning "atoning, expiating"; related to *piacula*, a noun meaning "sin offering," and to infinitive *piare*, meaning "to appease."

>   1. expiatory; atoning.

>   "The novitiate developed his own set of **piacular** acts he would perform until he could feel he had completed his essential rites of atonement."

>   2. culpable; wicked, requiring expiation.

>   "She was instilled with a sense of guilt in early childhood and often brooded over her **piacular** deeds."

>   Related words: **piacularly** (pī-AK-yə-lər-lee) *adverb;* **piacularness** (pī-AK-yə-lər-nis) *noun.*

picaresque (PIK-ə-RESK)
>   From Spanish *picaresco,* meaning "roguish."

>   resembling rogues; characterizing a type of fiction dealing with picaresque adventures.

>   "Many television shows, such as *The Mark of Zorro,* appealed to youngsters by centering about engaging fictional characters who weekly have **picaresque** encounters with their enemies."

>   Related words: **picara** (PIK-ər-ə), **picaro** (PIK-ə-ROH), and **picaroon** (PIK-ə-ROON) *all nouns.*

picayune (PIK-ə-YOON)
>   From Portuguese *picaioun,* from French *picaillon,* names of old copper coins of small value.

>   Also given as **picayunish** (PIK-ə-YOON-ish).

>   trifling, carping; mean, paltry.

>   "The new manager's criticism was mean-spirited and **picayune** rather than constructive."

>   Related words: **picayunishly** (PIK-ə-YOON-ish-lee) *adverb,* **picayunishness** (PIK-ə-YOON-ish-nis) *noun.*

piffling (PIF-ling)

    Origin uncertain.

    trifling, piddling; of little worth.

        "In organized baseball, intentionally throwing a bat is considered much more than a **piffling** act."

    Related word: **piffle** (PIF-əl) *noun* and *verb*.

pilose (PĪ-lohs)

    From Latin *pilosus*, meaning "hairy."

    Also given as **pilous** (PĪ-ləs)

    furry; covered with hair, especially soft hair.

        "Our pet had a **pilose** covering that made her fun to hold and stroke but always left behind handfuls of hair."

    Related word: **pilosity** (pī-LOS-i-tee) *noun*.

pinguid (PING-gwid)

    From Latin *pinguis*, from Greek *píon*, both meaning "fat, fertile."

    oily; abounding in fat.

        "My **pinguid** cuisine managed to fell so many victims that I have generally been excused from taking my turn at cooking for the entire crowd."

    Related word: **pinguidity** (ping-GWID-i-tee) *noun*.

piquant (PEE-kahnt)

    From French *piquant*, present participle of *piquer*, literally meaning "to prick"; generally interpreted as "to gall, irritate."

    1. of food: agreeably pungent or sharp of taste.

        "Almost everything he cooked, whether fish or fowl, was accented by a **piquant** sauce he had learned to prepare in the Far East."

    2. of wit, etc.: pleasantly provocative or stimulating.

        "Naomi was blessed with a **piquant** manner and good humor that enlivened any occasion."

    Related words: **piquantly** (PEE-kahnt-lee) *adverb*; **piquancy** (PEE-kahn-see) and **piquantness** (PEE-kahnt-nis) *both nouns*.

piteous (PIT-ee-əs)

    From Medieval Latin *pietosus*, from Latin *pietas*, both nouns meaning "a pity."

Also given as **pitiful** (PIT-i-fəl).

pathetic; deserving of pity; evoking pity.

"Once I had heard her **piteous** story from beginning to end, I resolved to give her all the help I could."

Related words: **piteously** (PIT-ee-əs-lee) *adverb*; **piteousness** (PIT-ee-əs-nis) *noun*.

pixilated (PIK-sə-LAY-tid)

Perhaps from American **pixie**, meaning "a sprite."

eccentric; mentally confused; fey, whimsical, silly.

"When once I had met the two old women, I decided they were charming but obviously **pixilated** and would need a watchful eye."

Related word: **pixilation** (PIK-sə-LAY-shən) *noun*.

placable (PLAYK-ə-bəl)

From Latin *placabilis*, from *placatus* past participle of *placare*, meaning "to calm, appease, reconcile."

Much better known in the negative, **implacable** (im-PLAYK-ə-bəl), translated as "unforgiving," says a great deal about our society.

forgiving; gentle, easily appeased.

"Strangely enough, the daughters of that harridan turned out to be entirely **placable** creatures and not at all like their mother."

Related words: **placabilitity** (PLAYK-ə-BIL-i-tee) and **placableness** (PLAYK-ə-bəl-nis) *both nouns*.

placatory (PLAY-kə-TOR-ee)

From Late Latin *placatorius*, meaning "appeasing, propitiatory"; from infinitive *placare*, meaning "to appease."

Also given as **placative** (PLAY-kə-tiv).

conciliatory; tending to placate.

"His initial response was entirely **placatory** and lulled us into thinking we were going to achieve the kind of resolution we all had hoped for."

Related words: **placate** (PLAY-kayt) *verb*; **placater** (PLAY-kayt-ər) and **placation** (play-KAY-shən) *both nouns*.

plangent (PLAN-jənt)

From Latin *plangens*, present participle of infinitive *plangere*, meaning "to beat the breast in grief; lament loudly."

loud sounding, especially with a mournful sound.

"The **plangent** church bell rang that Sunday with a somber, rarely heard sound, as though everyone knew we churchgoers had sad business ahead of us."

Related words: **plangently** (PLAN-jənt-lee) *adverb*; **plangency** (PLAN-jən-see) *noun*.

plethoric (ple-THOR-ik)

From Latin *plethoricus*, Greek *plethóra*, both meaning "fullness."

turgid; inflated, overfull; full to excess.

"In his speech the dean gave his usual **plethoric** masterpiece of eighteenth-century prose, unintentionally but effectively putting three hundred incoming freshmen to sleep."

Related words: **plethora** (PLETH-ər-ə) *noun*; **plethorically** (ple-THOR-i-kə-lee) *adverb*.

pluvious (PLOO-vee-əs)

From Latin *pluviosus*, meaning "rainy."

Also given as **pluvial** (PLOO-vee-əl).

rainy; pertaining to rain.

"We wondered how the town committee managed in each of the past ten years to select the only **pluvious** Saturday afternoon for our annual picnic in an otherwise parched month and to do so unerringly six months in advance."

Related word: **pluviosity** (PLOO-vee-OS-i-tee) *noun*.

pococurante (POH-koh-kuu-RAN-tee)

From Italian *poco*, meaning "little," + *curante*, present participle of *curare*, meaning "to care."

This adjective is more often used as a noun, meaning "a nonchalant person."

nonchalant; indifferent, caring little.

"After weeks of trying to get him to help us, we finally realized that he was **pococurante** and would never get involved."

Related words: **pococurantism** (POH-koh-kuu-RAN-tiz-əm) and **pococuranteism** (POH-koh-kuu-RAN-tee-iz-əm) *both nouns*.

porcine (POR-sīn)

From Latin *porcinus*, meaning "swinish; belonging to a hog."

piggish; swinish; resembling swine in appearance or manners; pertaining to swine.

"A **porcine** appearance was not at all what he had in mind when he decided to shave his face clean, yet that was what he saw when he looked into his mirror."

postprandial (pohst-PRAN-dee-əl)

From Latin *post-*, meaning "after," + *prandium*, meaning "lunch; a meal."

after a meal, especially after dinner.

"It did not take long for me to develop a physical need for a **postprandial** brandy or two, which soon was transformed into brandy without dinner."

Related word: **postprandially** (pohst-PRAN-dee-ə-lee) *adverb*.

See also **preprandial**.

pot-valiant (POT-VAL-yənt)

From English **pot,** meaning "container," and **valiant,** meaning "brave."

courageous only because of the support of alcoholic drink.

"When our **pot-valiant** platoon leader issued strong shots of whiskey at lunch before a night patrol, he surely knew what lay ahead of us."

Related words: **pot-valiantly** (POT-VAL-yənt-lee) *adverb*; **pot-valor** (POT-VAL-ər) and **pot-valiancy** (POT-VAL-yən-see) *both nouns*.

prandial (PRAN-dee-əl)

From Latin *prandium*, meaning "lunch" or "dinner."

See also **postprandial** and **preprandial**.

pertaining to a meal, especially dinner.

"Each time he went on the road, he was careful to make suitable notations in his diary for transportation, lodging, and **prandial** expenses."

Related word: **prandially** (PRAN-dee-ə-lee) *adverb*.

preceptive (pri-SEP-tiv)

From Latin *praeceptivus*, meaning "instructive, encouraging."

1. instructive; conveying information.

"Almost everything she publishes is intended to be entertaining but too often ends up being merely **preceptive**."

2. mandatory; conveying a command.

"Ownership of an automobile carries a responsibility to be aware of certain regulations and to follow their **preceptive** requirements."

Related words: **precept** (PREE-sept) *noun;* **preceptively** (pri-SEP-tiv-lee) *adverb.*

precipitate (pri-SIP-i-tit)

From Latin *praecipitatus,* past participle of infinitive *praecipitare,* meaning "to rush headlong; throw down."

Also given as **precipitative** (pri-SIP-i-TAY-tiv). *See also* **precipitous,** once a different word but now almost completely merged with **precipitate,** to no one's gain and purists' loss.

headlong; rushing onward; sudden, overhasty.

"Her parents believe Ella will surely have to pay for her **precipitate** decision to marry someone she had just met, but who knows whether she really made a mistake?"

Related words: **precipitately** (pri-SIP-i-tit-lee) *adverb;* **precipitateness** (pri-SIP-i-tit-nis), **precipitation** (pri-SIP-i-TAY-shən), and **precipitator** (pri-SIP-i-TAY-tər) *all nouns.*

precipitous (pri-SIP-i-təs)

From obsolete French *précipiteux,* meaning "dangerously steep."

Save **precipitous** for this meaning. Use **precipitate** for "sudden" and the like.

of terrain: dangerously steep or characterized by the presence of precipices.

"We would have made much better time if we had not been faced with so many **precipitous** rock slides that we had to ascend."

Related words: **precipitously** (pri-SIP-i-təs-lee) *adverb;* **precipitousness** (pri-SIP-i-təs-nis) *noun.*

predacious (pri-DAY-shəs)

From English **predatory,** from Latin *praedatorius,* meaning "marauding."

Also given as **predaceous.**

raptorial; rapacious, predatory.

"The biologist was concerned principally with investigating newborn goslings to learn how to protect them from **predacious** birds nesting nearby."

Related words: **predaciousness** (pri-DAY-shəs-nis) and **predacity** (pri-DAS-i-tee) *both nouns.*

prelapsarian (PREE-lap-SAIR-ee-ən)

From Latin *pre-*, prefix meaning "before," + *lapsus*, meaning "the fall." The fall, of course, was the original fall of mankind from virtue.

pertaining to any innocent period of life; occurring before the original fall from grace.

"What I liked best about the summer with our many grandchildren was the **prelapsarian** spirit they ebulliently showed in all their games."

preprandial (pree-PRAN-dee-əl)

For etymology, *see* **postprandial.**

before a meal, especially dinner.

"I was annoyed by her insistence that we all refrain from **preprandial** exercise, as though such exercise would hurt us in some way."

preternatural (PREE-tər-NACH-ər-əl)

From Latin phrase *praeter naturam*, meaning "beyond or outside nature."

supernatural; exceptional or abnormal.

"Fanny appeared to have a **preternatural** ability to hear the unexpressed thoughts of those near her."

Related words: **preternaturally** (PREE-tər-NACH-ə-rəl-ee) *adverb*; **preternaturalism** (PREE-tər-NACH-ə-rəl-iz-əm), **preternaturality** (PREE-tər-NACH-ə-RAL-i-tee), and **preternaturalness** (PREE-tər-NACH-ə-rəl-nis) *all nouns.*

proceleusmatic (PROS-ə-loos-MAT-ik)

From Greek *prokeleusmatikós*, meaning "incitement."

animating; inspiring; serving to inspire.

"Before the game, the band gave us a spirited, **proceleusmatic** rendition of the school song, but that did not prevent our first-string from losing the game without making a single hit."

procrustean (proh-KRUS-tee-ən)

From the name of the mythical robber *Procrustes*, who cruelly stretched the limbs of a captured traveler to make them fit the length of his bed.

tending to produce uniformity by violent and arbitrary means.

"Our leader assured compliance within his staff by assigning the most savage and loyal of his soldiers to employ **procrustean** methods in enforcing his peremptory orders."

prolegomenous (PROH-li-GOM-ə-nəs)
From Greek *prolegómenon*, meaning "saying beforehand."

prefatory; introductory; especially, given to making tedious opening remarks.

"Edward knew his mother was warming up to deliver a stern rebuke when she would clear her throat audibly and then launch into one of her favorite **prolegomenous** attacks before finally announcing the punishment she had already selected."

Related words: **prolegomenon** (PROH-li-GOM-ə-NON) *singular noun*; **prolegomena** (PROH-li-GOM-ə-nah) *plural noun*.

prolix (proh-LIKS)
From Latin *prolixus*, meaning "long, wide, extended."

1. of speech or writing: verbose, wordy; overly long.

"By May I was gratified to find that many students had learned to prune their **prolix** sentences."

2. of a person: given to verbosity or wordiness.

"It seems that **prolix** neighbors never miss a chance to catch me and won't stop talking when I'm in a hurry."

Related words: **prolixly** (proh-LIKS-lee) *adverb*; **prolixity** (proh-LIK-si-tee) *noun*.

propitious (prə-PISH-əs)
From Latin *propitius*, meaning "favorable, gracious"; from infinitive *petere*, meaning "to aim at, attack."

auspicious; favorable, presenting favorable conditions.

"Everyone agreed that conditions were **propitious** for starting a new dot.com, in fact for starting any new enterprise."

Related words: **propitiously** (prə-PISH-əs-lee) *adverb*; **propitiousness** (prə-PISH-əs-nis) *noun*.

protean (PROH-tee-ən)
From the name *Proteus*, the mythical god who could prophesy and could change his shape at will.

variable in form; assuming at will various forms or characters.

"Voters appear to have punished the governor for his **protean** positions on important matters of public interest."

Related word: **proteanism** (PROH-tee-ə-niz-əm) *noun.*

prurient (PRUUR-ee-ənt)

From Latin *pruriens*, present participle of *prurire*, meaning "to itch, be wanton."

given to lewd thoughts; impure-minded.

"Our **prurient** public censor has confessed to spending much of his office time poring over magazines featuring photographs of nude men and women and advertising collections of similar photographs."

Related words: **pruriently** (PRUUR-ee-ənt-lee) *adverb;* **prurience** (PRUUR-ee-əns) and **pruriency** (PRUUR-ee-en-see) *both nouns.*

puerperal (pyoo-UR-pər-əl)

From Neo-Latin *puerperalis*, meaning "of childbirth"; from Latin *puerperium*, meaning "childbirth."

accompanied by or resulting from childbirth.

"My sister-in-law's case of **puerperal** fever was quickly cured after application of modern antibiotics."

pusillanimous (PYOO-sə-LAN-ə-məs)

From Late Latin *pusillus*, meaning "paltry," + *animus*, meaning "disposition."

cowardly; fainthearted; lacking resolution; manifesting cowardliness.

"The **pusillanimous** measures of the administration were met with almost universal condemnation."

Related words: **pusillanimously** (PYOO-sə-LAN-ə-məs-lee) *adverb;* **pusillanimity** (PYOO-sə-lə-NIM-i-tee) *noun.*

putative (PYOO-tə-tiv)

From Late Latin *putativus*, from Latin *putatus*, past participle of *putare*, meaning "to suppose."

reputed, supposed; commonly regarded as so by reputation.

"After months of dreary and repetitious courtroom argument, Albert was seen as the **putative** winner of the hard-fought case."

Related word: **putatively** (PYOO-tə-tiv-lee) *adverb.*

putrescible (pyoo-TRES-ə-bəl)

From Latin infinitive *putrescere*, meaning "to grow rotten."

Also given as **putrescent** (pyoo-TRES-ənt).

liable to rot or become putrid.

"The **putrescible** odor told me that the vegetables were on the verge and I'd better throw them out."

Related words: **putrefy** (PYOO-trə-FĪ) *verb*; **putrefaction** (PYOO-trə-FAK-shən), **putrescence** (pyoo-TRES-əns), **putrescency** (pyoo-TRES-ən-see), and **putrescibility** (pyoo-TRES-i-BIL-i-tee) *all nouns*.

quadrennial (kwo-DREN-ee-əl)

From Latin *quadriennium,* meaning "four years."

Also given as **quadriennial** (KWOD-ree-EN-ee-əl).

1. occurring every fourth year.

   "The **quadrennial** election was almost at hand, affecting almost all political decisions that had to be made."

2. lasting for four years.

   "The chairman knew that a **quadrennial** budget would have to be formulated and voted upon before the new term."

   Related words: **quadrennium** (kwo-DREN-ee-əm) and **quadriennium** (KWOD-ree-EN-ee-əm) *both nouns.*

qualmish (KWAH-mish)

From English **qualm,** meaning "compunction," + **-ish,** meaning "inclined to." The source of **qualm** is unknown.

1. apt to have uneasy feelings or pangs of conscience.

   "Her recent unfortunate experiences have left Ellen **qualmish** about doing anything to help our cause."

2. apt to cause uneasy feelings.

   "No matter what I told the committee chairman about the secret intentions of the minority, he would do nothing to disturb their **qualmish** plans."

3. nauseated.

"Without fail, every time our ship leaves port I immediately feel **qualmish** even though I have never actually become sick to my stomach."

Related words: **qualmishly** (KWAH-mish-lee) *adverb;* **qualm** (kwahm) and **qualmishness** (KWAH-mish-nis) *both nouns.*

quaquaversal (KWAY-kwə-VUR-səl)

From Latin *quaqua*, literally meaning "whatever way," + versus, meaning "toward"; together meaning "turned everywhere."

Although this seldom-encountered word is a legitimate part of the English lexicon, it is included here primarily to show that our glorious language has a word for every situation.

of a geological formation: dipping down from the center in all directions.

"At the presumed top of the universe, you are said to find a **quaquaversal** pinnacle large enough to stand upon even though the conception is anything but real."

Related word: **quaquaversally** (KWAY-kwue-VUR-sə-lee) *adverb.*

queasy (KWEE-zee)

Possibly from Middle English *qweisy* or *coisy*, meaning "uneasy."

1. of persons: liable to become sick; feeling nausea; uneasy, feeling uncomfortable.

"My youngest granddaughter says the only thing she doesn't like about our local diner is that she feels **queasy** after she eats there."

2. nauseating; tending to cause nausea.

"Ann thinks she is clever when she combines heterogeneous leftovers of any origin in a **queasy** glop that she calls soup."

Related words: **queasily** (KWEE-zi-lee) *adverb;* **queasiness** (KWEE-zi-nis) *noun.*

quercine (KWUR-sĭn)

From Latin *quercus*, meaning "oak tree" + *-ine*, an adjectival suffix.

made of oak, oaken.

"Our **quercine** staircase was admired by all those who saw it, but my wife and I were always aware of the squeaks it gave off at every step."

querulous (KWER-ə-ləs)

From Latin *querulus*, meaning "complaining; plaintive."

1. given to complaining; full of complaints.

"Whenever we visited my **querulous** aunt, she regaled us with blow-by-blow accounts of terrible experiences she enjoyed."

2. peevish; uttered in complaint.

"Fred's **querulous** admonitions were too frequent and too unvarying to be taken seriously."

Related words: **querulously** (KWER-ə-ləs-lee) *adverb*; **querulousness** (KWER-ə-ləs-nis) *noun*.

quiescent (kwee-ES-ənt)

From Latin *quiescens*, present participle of infinitive *quiescere*, meaning "to keep quiet; be at peace."

motionless; at rest, inactive.

"The **quiescent** state a wounded soldier must exhibit to evade capture by enemy troops was more than I bargained for."

Related words: **quiescently** (kwee-ES-ənt-lee) *adverb*; **quiescence** (kwee-ES-əns) and **quiescency** (kwee-ES-ən-see) *both nouns.*

quixotic (kwik-SOT-ik)

From the name of the visionary hero of *Don Quixote* by Cervantes.

Also given as **quixotical** (kwik-SOT-i-kəl).

1. of a person: resembling the personality of Quixote, therefore striving with enthusiasm for visionary ideals.

"There was no way to convert his **quixotic** idealism into realistic goals that would enable him to raise his income substantially."

2. impractical; impulsive, rashly unpredictable.

"It was difficult to convince our **quixotic** leader that swimming miles across the bay after darkness was not feasible, since he was not an experienced distance swimmer."

Related words: **quixotically** (kwik-SOT-i-kəl-ee) *adverb*; **quixotism** (KWIK-sə-TIZ-əm) *noun.*

quotidian (kwoh-TID-ee-ən)

From Latin *quotidianus*, also given as *cottidianus*, meaning "daily, everyday, ordinary."

daily, everyday; ordinary, commonplace.

"Wednesday began as a day like all other days: on his desk lay the **quotidian** head counts arranged by departments with totals and subtotals supplied, even though he could not recall why he had asked for them in the first place."

Related words: **quotidianly** (kwoh-TID-ee-ən-lee) *adverb*; **quotidianness** (kwoh-TID-ee-ən-nis) *noun*.

R

rabid (RAB-id)

From Latin *rabidus*, meaning "raving, mad, impetuous"; from infinitive *rabere*, meaning "to rave."

1. furious, raging; violent in nature or opinion.

"There are **rabid** baseball fans and there are **rabid** Yankee fans, the latter being irrational forms of the former."

2. afflicted with rabies—an infectious disease formerly called hydrophobia.

"If your pet has been properly inoculated, chances are it will probably never be **rabid**."

Related words: **rabidly** (RAB-id-lee) *adverb*; **rabidity** (rə-BID-i-tee) and **rabidness** (RAB-id-nis) *both nouns*.

raffish (RAF-ish)

From English **raff**, said to be from **riffraff**, meaning "common people; rabble."

1. tawdry; vulgar, cheap.

"She knew her coworkers considered her manner of dress **raffish**, but she would not change, saying she felt comfortable in her ways."

2. engagingly disreputable.

"He had the **raffish** good looks that wealthy middle-aged women apparently found attractive."

Related words: **raffishly** (RAF-ish-lee) *adverb*; **raffishness** (RAF-ish-nis) *noun*.

rakish (RAY-kish)

From English **rake,** meaning "a profligate, licentious, wild person."

of one's appearance: smart, jaunty, dashing.

"Most of all it was the newcomer's **rakish** hat and affected walking stick combined with a swagger that made him the darling of women but unacceptable among men his own age."

Related words: **rakishly** (RAY-kish-lee) *adverb;* **rakishness** (RAY-kish-nis) *noun.*

rambunctious (ram-BUNGK-shəs)

A word of uncertain origin.

of persons and encounters: uncontrollable, boisterous, noisy.

"Once it became clear unlimited hard liquor was free for the asking, the party was sure to become **rambunctious** and end unpredictably, so our friends left as soon as possible."

Related words: **rambunctiously** (ram-BUNGK-shəs-lee) *adverb;* **rambunctiousness** (ram-BUNGK-shəs-nis) *noun.*

rancorous (RANG-kər-əs)

From English **rancor,** meaning "malice," from Latin adjective *rancens,* meaning "putrid."

venomous; full of resentment; showing ill feeling.

"So **rancorous** was his envy, so sharp the wound he suffered, that he could not bear even to look at his opponent."

Related words: **rancorously** (RANG-kər-əs-lee) *adverb;* **rancorousness** (RANG-kər-əs-nis) *noun.*

rapacious (rə-PAY-shəs)

From Latin *rapax,* meaning "greedy, grasping, ravenous"; from *rapere,* infinitive meaning "to seize, carry off by force."

The infamous verb "to rape" is scarcely able to hide its origins.

1. predatory; exceptionally greedy, extortionate.

"It was shocking to find that the **rapacious** burglars did not overlook even the tiniest gem in her pathetic collection."

2. given to seizing for the satisfaction of greed.

"She practiced a **rapacious** management style that landed her in deep trouble with antitrust laws."

Related words: **rapaciously** (rə-PAY-shəs-lee) *adverb*; **rapacity** (rə-PAS-i-tee) and **rapaciousness** (rə-PAY-shəs-nis) *both nouns.*

raunchy (RAWN-chee)
Of uncertain origin.

vulgar, smutty, dirty; lecherous, suggestive.

"The comedian's **raunchy** stories actually seemed to offend some persons, but most of his audience found them very funny and gave his career a big boost."

Related words: **raunchily** (RAWN-chi-lee) *adverb*; **raunch** (rawnch) and **raunchiness** (RAWN-chee-nis) *both nouns.*

rebarbative (ree-BAHR-bə-tiv)
From French feminine adjective *rébarbative*—masculine *rébarbatif*—meaning "unprepossessing, repellent, unattractive"; from *rébarber*, meaning "to be unattractive," and from French *barbe* and Latin *barba*, both meaning "beard."

As the synonyms for beard come to mind, think how beards once made the man and how since then these hairy appurtenances have gone in and out of style.

unattractive, dull; forbidding; causing aversion; unpleasant, objectionable.

"His friends, always willing to stand firm in their decisiveness, said his **rebarbative** personality matched his homely face."

Related words: **rebarbatively** (ree-BAHR-bə-tiv-lee) *adverb*; **rebarbativity** (ree-BAHR-bə-TIV-i-tee) and **rebarbativeness** (ree-BAHR-bə-tiv-nis) *both nouns.*

recalcitrant (ri-KAL-si-trənt)
From *recalcitrans*, present participle of infinitive *recalcitrare*, meaning "to kick back."

refractory; obstinately disobedient; difficult to manage.

"The novice teacher was at wit's end trying to find a solution to the problem of how to handle **recalcitrant** students."

Related words: **recalcitrancy** (ri-KAL-si-trən-see) and **recalcitrance** (ri-KAL-si-trəns) *both nouns.*

recherché (rə-SHAIR-shay)
From French past participle of infinitive *rechercher*, meaning "to search for assiduously."

carefully sought after; arcane, choice, rare; pretentious.

"The antiques dealer's apartment proved astonishing, full of the most **recherché** treasures the young couple had ever seen."

recondite (REK-ən-DĪT)

From Latin *reconditus*, past participle of infinitive *recondere*, meaning "to hide, put away."

abstruse; deep, profound; esoteric; obscure.

"It was almost a year after my illness had passed before I began to recover my strength and became able to resume my **recondite** research."

Related words: **reconditely** (REK-ən-DĪT-lee) *adverb*; **reconditeness** (REK-ən-DĪT-nis) *noun*.

recumbent (ri-KUM-bənt)

From Latin *recumbens*, present participle of infinitive *recumbere*, meaning "to lie down, recline; sink down."

lying down; reclining; prostrate; leaning; idle.

"When I first saw her at the beach, she was **recumbent** and seemed unwilling to stir herself even though she was obviously getting a bad burn."

Related words: **recumbently** (ri-KUM-bənt-lee) *adverb*; **recumbency** (ri-KUM-bən-see) and **recumbence** (ri-KUM-bəns) *both nouns*.

redivivus (RED-ə-VEE-vəs)

From Latin *redivivus*, meaning "renovated, revived."

An example of a Latin word taken into English without change.

revived; living again; come back to life.

"From the way that new pitcher throws, he's Christy Mathewson **redivivus** or I don't know the first thing about baseball."

redolent (RED-l-ənt)

From the present participle of the Latin infinitive *redolere*, meaning "to give off a smell, smell of."

fragrant; smelling; reminiscent.

"When I first entered the sitting room, which was so **redolent** of jasmine, it seemed for a moment I had entered a different culture."

Related words: **redolently** (RED-l-ənt-lee) *adverb*; **redolence** (RED-l-əns) and **redolency** (RED-l-ən-see) *both nouns.*

redoubtable (ri-DOW-tə-bəl)

From French *redoutable,* meaning "formidable, terrible."

formidable; to be feared; evoking respect.

"From the way the new president acted at the meeting it was obvious that this **redoubtable** man would soon have his problems under control."

Related words: **redoubted** (ri-DOW-tid) *adjective;* **redoubtably** (ri-DOW-tə-blee) *adverb;* **redoubtableness** (ri-DOW-tə-bəl-nis) *noun.*

refractory (ri-FRAK-tə-ree)

From Latin *refractarius,* meaning "obstinate, stubborn."

unmanageable; stubborn, perverse, rebellious.

"It was clear the **refractory** child represented much more than an ordinary case of disobedience and would have to be treated with the greatest of care and professional skill."

Related words: **refractorily** (ri-FRAK-tə-rə-lee) *adverb;* **refractoriness** (ri-FRAK-tə-ree-nis) *noun.*

refulgent (ri-FUL-jənt)

From Latin *refulgens,* present participle of *refulgere,* meaning "to flash back, radiate light."

radiant; resplendent, shining brightly; reflecting a brilliant light.

"Although the woman's jewelry was demonstrably fake, it had been made so skillfully that its **refulgent** brilliance was dazzling."

Related words: **refulgently** (ri-FUL-jənt-lee) *adverb;* **refulgence** (ri-FUL-jəns), **refulgency** (ri-FUL-jən-see), and **refulgentness** (ri-FUL-jənt-nis) *all nouns.*

relevant (REL-ə-vənt)

From Latin *relevans,* present participle of infinitive *relevare,* meaning "to lift up, lighten; comfort."

pertinent; bearing on the matter at hand.

"My students were informed at the start of the term that they could always say anything they wanted as long as their remarks were **relevant** to subjects under discussion at the time."

Related words: **relevantly** (REL-ə-vənt-lee) *adverb*; **relevance** (REL-ə-vəns) and **relevancy** (REL-ə-vən-see) *both nouns.*

renitent (REN-i-tənt)

From Latin *renitens* present participle of infinitive *reniti*, meaning "to struggle, resist."

recalcitrant; opposing assiduously; resistant, resisting pressure.

"Despite his determinedly **renitent** stance, he found himself unable to overcome the council's pressure to oust him."

Related words: **renitence** (REN-i-təns) and **renitency** (REN-i-tən-see) *both nouns.*

reprobate (REP-rə-BAYT)

From Latin *reprobatus*, past participle of infinitive *reprobare*, meaning "to reprove."

Also given as a noun and as the adjective *reprobative* (REP-rə-BAY-tiv).

morally depraved; unprincipled; beyond hope of salvation.

"He was pleased to find that the club would not tolerate **reprobate** conduct and had recently blackballed prospective members when they were found to have less than impeccable reputations."

Related words: **reprobation** (REP-rə-BAY-shən), **reprobacy** (REP-rə-bə-see), and **reprobateness** (REP-rə-BAYT-nis), *all nouns.*

retroussé (RE-troo-SAY)

From French past participle of *retrousser*, meaning "to turn up."

said especially of the nose: turned up.

"Undoubtedly there are some who think a **retroussé** nose indicates a person of spunk."

riant (REE-ənt)

From French *riant*, present participle of *rire*, meaning "to laugh"; from Latin *ridere*, with the same meaning.

Also given as **rident** (RĪD-nt).

cheerful; laughing, smiling; gay.

"Ruth is a happy child, almost always **riant** in demeanor, loving to tell and hear jokes."

Related word: **riantly** (REE-ənt-lee) *adverb.*

rinky-dink (RING-kee-DINGK)
Slang; origin unknown.

worthless; outmoded, generally inferior.

"He was advised to seek employment only at reputable companies with solid financial statements and to avoid **rinky-dink** companies promising rosy futures for their new staff members."

risible (RIZ-ə-bəl)
From Late Latin *risibilis*, meaning "laughable"; from Latin infinitive *ridere*, meaning "to laugh."

ludicrous; comical; pertaining to laughter; given to laughter.

"Buster Keaton's silent movies may have been intended only to be **risible**, but they were also ingeniously perceptive of human motivations."

Related word: **risibility** (RIZ-ə-BIL-i-tee) *noun.*

ritzy (RIT-see)
From the name of the sumptuous hotels operated by César Ritz, a Swiss hotelier of the early twentieth century.

posh; elegant; fashionable and luxurious.

"Not only did he insist on staying at **ritzy** hotels, but he ran up enormous bills for room service meals for his friends and himself."

Related words: **ritzily** (RITS-i-lee) *adverb*; **ritziness** (RITS-i-nis) *noun.*

robustious (roh-BUS-chəs)
From English **robust**, meaning "vigorous," + **-ious**, an adjectival suffix.

robust, boisterous; rough, strong.

"The table was dominated by six **robustious** frontiersmen who, to my great relief, had been required by the management to remove and surrender their firearms before the game could begin."

Related word: **robustiously** (roh-BUS-chəs-lee) *adverb.*

rubescent (roo-BES-ənt)
From Latin *rubescens*, present participle of infinitive *rubescere*, meaning "to redden, blush"; from *ruber*, meaning "red."

blushing; tending to redness.

"Hank's only problem when playing poker was his incurably **rubescent** visage, which forever was the tip-off to a winning hand he was holding."

Related word: **rubescence** (roo-BES-əns) *noun.*

rubicund (ROO-bi-KUND)

From Latin *rubicundus,* meaning "red, ruddy"; from *ruber,* meaning "red."

reddish; flushed, inclined to redness attributed to good living.

"Zane's **rubicund** good looks apparently masked years of high living, which finally took their toll when he died at fifty-five."

Related word: **rubicundity** (ROO-bi-KUN-di-tee) *noun.*

ruthful (ROOTH-fəl)

From Middle English *ruthe,* meaning "pity, regret."

The English word **ruthful** is almost never heard, in contrast with **ruthless** — meaning "cruel, without compassion" — which rears its head every day.

compassionate; sorrowful; causing sorrow; feeling remorse.

"It was Ron's way to suppress any tendency to feel **ruthful** about conditions he could neither understand nor repair."

Related words: **ruthfully** (ROOTH-fə-lee) *adverb;* **ruthfulness** (ROOTH-fəl-nis) *noun.*

ruthless. *See* **ruthful**.

rutilant (ROOT-l-nt)

From Latin *rutilans,* present participle of infinitive *rutilare,* meaning "to glow red, color red"; from *rutilus,* meaning "reddish, golden, shining."

scintillating with golden or reddish light; shining, gleaming, glittering.

"Her living room, ready for the Christmas season, was **rutilant** with beautiful colored lights."

S

sabulous (SAB-yə-ləs)

From Latin *sabulosus*, meaning "sandy"; from *sabulum*, meaning "sand."

'Swonderful, 'sfabulous was a songwriter's tribute to Hollywood love, but **sabulous** is the unwelcome adornment you take on at a beach.

arenaceous (a geologist's term); sandy; consisting of sand.

"Lenny thought it extraordinary that his **sabulous** property on Long Island, nothing more than a small mountain of sand, ended 'only a few miles from Europe,' as he put it."

Related word: **sabulosity** (SAB-yə-LOS-i-tee) *noun.*

saccadic (sa-KAHD-ik)

From English **saccade** (sa-KAHD), meaning "a jerky movement."

jerky; characterized by discontinuous movement.

"I finally had a chance to use a camera capable of photographing the **saccadic** movements made by the eyes during reading."

sacerdotal (SAS-ər-DOHT-əl)

From Latin *sacerdotalis*, from *sacerdotium*, meaning "priesthood."

Often mispronounced by semiliterate pretenders as though it were spelled *sacridotal.*

priestly; befitting a priest.

"The **sacerdotal** robes worn during the ordination of several cardinals were ornate and heavy, entirely befitting the gravity of the occasion."

Related words: **sacerdotally** (SAS-ər-DOH-tə-lee) *adverb*; **sacerdotalism** (SAS-ər-DOH-tə-LIZ-əm) and **sacerdotalist** (SAS-ər-DOHT-əl-ist) *both nouns.*

sacrilegious (SAK-rə-LEE-jəs)

From Middle English *sacrilegiose*, from Latin *sacrilegium*, from *sacrilegus*, meaning "one who steals sacred things."

The adjective **sacrilegious** should not be confused with the adjective **religious** either in pronunciation or in definition.

pertaining to the profaning of anything sacred; guilty of stealing such things.

"When you go there, be mindful of local customs lest you say or do something considered **sacrilegious**."

Related words: **sacrilegiously** (SAK-rə-LEE-jəs-lee) *adverb*; **sacrilege** (SAK-rə-lij) and **sacrilegiousness** (SAK-rə-LEE-jəs-nis) *both nouns.*

sacrosanct (SAK-rə-SANGKT)

From Latin *sacrosanctus*, meaning "inviolable," from *sacro sanctus*, meaning "made holy by sacred rite."

1. sacred, inviolable; secured by a religious sanction from violation or infringement.

"The old city was finally declared **sacrosanct** and from then on was considered safe against any modern encroachment."

2. beyond criticism or change.

"Dora thought her parents' way of doing things was **sacrosanct** and was offended by any suggestion of improvement."

Related words: **sacrosanctness** (SAK-rə-SANGKT-nis) and **sacrosanctity** (SAK-rə-SANGK-ti-tee) *both nouns.*

sagacious (sə-GAY-shəs)

From English **sagacity**, from Latin *sagacitas*, both meaning "wisdom."

shrewd, having exceptional mental discernment.

"Harry clearly was the more **sagacious** of the two lawyers, but he lacked the ability to take on a task and see it through to completion."

Related words: **sagaciously** (sə-GAY-shəs-lee) *adverb*; **sagacity** (sə-GAS-i-tee) and **sagaciousness** (sə-GAY-shəs-nis) *both nouns.*

salacious (sə-LAY-shəs)

From Latin *salax*, meaning "lustful"; from infinitive *salire*, meaning "to leap, spring, throb."

lecherous, lustful; obscene.

"Readers of **salacious** novels were said once upon a time to have disguised their reading matter in plain brown wrappers."

Related words: **salaciously** (sə-LAY-shəs-lee) *adverb*; **salaciousness** (sə-LAY-shəs-nis) and **salacity** (sə-LAS-i-tee) *both nouns.*

salubrious (sə-LOO-bree-əs)

From Latin *salubris*, meaning "health-giving, wholesome"; from *salus*, meaning "health, welfare."

Also given as **salutary**, which see.

healthful; conducive to health.

"The prescribed diet is undeniably **salubrious**, yet one might hope for something more appetizing."

Related words: **salubriously** (sə-LOO-bree-əs-lee) *adverb*; **salubriousness** (sə-LOO-bree-əs-nis) *noun.*

salutary (SAL-yə-TER-ee)

From Latin *salutaris*, meaning "wholesome, healthy, beneficial"; from *salus*, meaning "health, welfare."

Also given as **salubrious**.

healthful; wholesome; promoting health.

"Many physicians recommend a regime of moderate exercise and carefully selected diet among other things as a **salutary** style of living."

Related words: **salutarily** (SAL-yə-TER-ə-lee) *adverb*; **salutariness** (SAL-yə-TER-ə-nis) *noun.*

sanguinary (SANG-gwə-NER-ee)

From Latin *sanguinarius*, meaning "bloodthirsty, pertaining to blood."

Not to be confused with **sanguine**, which see.

bloody; bloodthirsty; marked with blood; delighting in carnage; characterized by slaughter.

"The famous general was portrayed cinematically as a person who reveled in **sanguinary** military encounters."

Related words: **sanguinarily** (SANG-gwə-NER-i-lee) *adverb*; **san-guinariness** (SANG-gwə-NER-ee-nis) *noun.*

sanguine (SANG-gwin)

From Latin *sanguineus,* meaning "bloody"; from *sanguis,* meaning "blood."

Notice that the synonyms supplied do not give license to use **san-guinary** as an alternative for **sanguine,** which means "optimistic" or "ruddy."

1. cheerfully optimistic; hopeful, confident.

"Edwina may not be **sanguine** about her chance to land the cov-eted job, but she has certainly not given up hope."

2. ruddy; reddish.

"Alice's **sanguine** cheeks fool her family into thinking she is health-ier than her friends, when the fact is she has a physical problem that causes her high color."

Related words: **sanguinely** (SANG-gwin-lee) *adverb*; **sanguinness** (SANG-gwin-nis) and **sanguinity** (sang-GWIN-i-tee) *both nouns*; **sanguineous** (sang-GWIN-ee-əs), **sanguinolent** (sang-GWIN-ə-lənt), and **sanguivorous** (sang-GWIV-ər-əs) *all adjectives.*

saporific (SAP-ə-RIF-ik)

From Neo-Latin *saporificus,* meaning "tasty"; from *sapor,* meaning "taste."

Notice that **saporific** bears no relationship to **soporific** (SOP-ə-RIF-ik), an adjective that means "causing sleep." *See* **soporiferous.**

imparting flavor, producing flavor.

"The directions his books supply for preparing most dishes neglect the spices needed by anyone who wants to achieve **saporific** results."

Related words: **saporous** (SAP-ər-əs) *adjective*; **saporosity** (SAP-ə-ROS-i-tee) and **sapor** (SAY-pər) *both nouns.*

sardonic (sahr-DON-ik)

From Latin *sardonius,* from Greek *sardónios,* both meaning "of Sar-dinia."

Lest you think you have to be in on a Sardinian joke known only to a few, read on. Old botany textbooks suggest that any of the bitter plants that grow in Sardinia produce in hapless diners a painful grimace that is accompanied by convulsions of laughter and eventual death. Are these the first recorded instances of persons who laughed themselves to death?

sneering, cynical; bitter, scornful, mocking.

"The lecturer's **sardonic** manner intimidated his students."

Related words: **sardonically** (sahr-DON-i-kə-lee) *adverb*; **sardonicism** (sahr-DON-ə-SIZ-əm) *noun*.

scathing (SKAY-*th*ing)

From English **scathe,** meaning "to criticize harshly."

searing; severe; injurious.

"Donald Ross, your freshman writing instructor, doesn't seem to understand that his **scathing** public criticisms of the classes' papers wound the writers and do not teach."

Related words: **scathe** (skay*th*) *verb*; **scatheless** (SKAY*TH*-lis) *adjective*; **scathelessly** (SKAY*TH*-lis-lee) and **scathingly** (SKAY*TH*-ing-lee) *both adverbs*.

scilicet (SIL-ə-SET)

From Latin *scilicet,* short for *scire licet,* literally meaning "it is permitted to know." **Scilicet** is usually abbreviated as **sc.** or as **scil.**

namely; that is to say; to wit; evidently, of course.

"I believe there were three principal reasons why the German navy did not invade Great Britain during World War II, **sc.** the British army, the British air force, and the British navy."

scrofulous (SKROF-yə-ləs)

From English **scrofula,** meaning "a type of tuberculosis," + **-ous,** an adjectival suffix meaning "full of."

morally corrupt; affected with scrofula.

"The prudish teacher would not accept reports on any books she considered **scrofulous.**"

Related words: **scrofulously** (SKROF-yə-ləs-lee) *adverb*; **scrofula** (SKROF-yə-lə) and **scrofulousness** (SKROF-yə-ləs-nis) *both nouns*.

scurrilous (SKUR-ə-ləs)

From English **scurrile,** an archaic word from Latin *scurrilis,* meaning "jeering"; from Latin *scurra,* meaning "buffoon; dandy."

of language or behavior: coarsely opprobrious; obscenely abusive.

"After one semester away from home, Jeanette had acquired the entire **scurrilous** vocabulary of a drunken sailor on shore leave."

Related words: **scurrilously** (SKUR-ə-ləs-lee) *adverb*; **scurrilous- ness** (SKUR-ə-ləs-nis) and **scurrility** (skə-RIL-i-tee) *both nouns*.

sedulous (SEJ-ə-ləs)
From Latin *sedulus*, meaning "careful, assiduous, diligent."

1. of actions: persistent, constant.

"The company no longer was known for the **sedulous** attention to customers' welfare that had put it on the map."

2. of persons: diligent, persistent, assiduous.

"Professor Thirlwall was known as a **sedulous** scholar whose writ- ings were clear, concise, and authoritative."

Related words: **sedulously** (SEJ-ə-ləs-lee) *adverb*; **sedulousness** (SEJ-ə-ləs-nis) and **sedulity** (si-DOO-li-tee) *both nouns*.

sempiternal (SEM-pi-TUR-nəl)
From Late Latin *sempiternalis*, from Latin *sempiternus*, meaning "everlasting."

as a literary word: everlasting: enduring constantly and continually.

"We were treated to the most exciting of dinners, featuring various patés, the clearest of broths, and the **sempiternal** English roast beef."

Related word: **sempiternally** (SEM-pi-TUR-nə-lee) *adverb*.

senescent (si-NES-ənt)
From Latin *senescens*, present participle of the infinitive *senescere*, meaning "to grow old."

growing old; elderly.

"When Lawrence heard that his children considered him **senes- cent** and fit only for life in a rest home, he packed his few things and moved to his country retreat, there to be alone until the end of his life."

Related word: **senescence** (si-NES-əns) *noun*.

sensual (SEN-shoo-əl)
From Latin *sensualis* from *sensus*, meaning "sense, sensation."

Compare **sensual** with **sensuous**.

carnal; fleshly; worldly, materialistic; lewd, unchaste; inclined to gratification of the senses.

"Suddenly free of the puritanical constraints of home, Hastings indulged in the **sensual** temptations of his new environment."

Related words: **sensualism** (SEN-shoo-ə-LIZ-əm), **sensualist** (SEN-shoo-ə-list), **sensuality** (SEN-shoo-AL-i-tee), and **sensualization** (SEN-shoo-əl-i-ZAY-shən) *all nouns.*

sensuous (SEN-shoo-əs)

From Latin *sensus,* meaning "sense."

This adjective refers to communication, not to carnal instincts. Compare **sensuous** with **sensual.**

received through one or more senses; pertaining to the senses.

"The aroma of the fruit, the color and shape of the vegetables, the cries of the merchants hawking their offerings—all these made shopping for dinner a **sensuous** adventure."

Related words: **sensuously** (SEN-shoo-əs-lee) *adverb;* **sensuousness** (SEN-shoo-əs-nis) and **sensuosity** (SEN-shoo-OS-i-tee) *both nouns.*

sententious (sen-TEN-shəs)

From Latin *sententiosus,* meaning "pithy; meaningful."

1. of a person: self-righteous; given to pompous moralizing or to overuse of pithy maxims; putting on an air of wisdom.

"He fancied himself an eloquent wise man, but the **sententious** ex-senator actually was nothing more than a tedious windbag."

2. of writing: self-righteous; abounding in aphorisms or maxims; dull and moralizing.

"His writing style was **sententious,** full of old saws and gratuitous advice."

Related words: **sententiously** (sen-TEN-shəs-lee) *adverb;* **sententiousness** (sen-TEN-shəs-nis) and **sententiosity** (sen-TEN-shee-OS-i-tee) *both nouns.*

sentient (SEN-shənt)

From Latin *sentiens,* present participle of infinitive *sentire,* meaning "to feel."

conscious; having the power of perception by the senses.

"A **sentient** individual cannot fail to understand the signs of imminent warfare and what armed conflict will eventually mean to all of us."

Related words: **sentiently** (SEN-shənt-lee) *adverb*; **sentience** (SEN-shəns) *noun*.

serendipitous (SER-ən-DIP-i-təs)

From English **serendipity**, meaning "luck," based on *Serendip*, an ancient name of Ceylon, today called Sri Lanka.

Coinage of **serendipitous** is credited to the eighteenth-century English novelist Horace Walpole, who published a fairy tale called "The Three Princes of Serendip," telling of three princes who were always discovering things they had not been looking for. And this is the heart of **serendipity** and its adjective **serendipitous**.

1. fortuitous; found by accident.

"The prospectors made their **serendipitous** discovery of gold in the mountains of California."

2. beneficial; favorable; welcome.

"Many of the century's **serendipitous** chemical innovations can be attributed to nothing more than chance and a willingness to work day and night."

Related words: **serendipitously** (SER-ən-DIP-i-təs-lee) *adverb*; **serendipity** (SER-ən-DIP-i-tee), **serendipiter** (SER-ən-DIP-i-tər), **serendipitist** (SER-ən-DIP-i-tist), and **serendipper** (SER-ən-DIP-ər) *all nouns*.

simplistic (sim-PLIS-tik)

From English **simple,** a word that is well understood.

Simplistic, on the other hand, is one of the words that bedevil people who fail to understand its correct use in English.

oversimplified.

"One great danger is to approach a very complex problem with a **simplistic** solution in mind."

Related words: **simplistically** (sim-PLIS-ti-kə-lee) *adverb*; **simplism** (SIM-pliz-əm) *noun*.

sinistrous (SIN-ə-strəs)

From Latin *sinister*, meaning "left, on the left hand"; also, as one might expect, "perverse, unfavorable."

Also given as **sinistral** (SIN-ə-strəl).

Now you can understand why our superstitious society traditionally has been less than fair with left-handed persons.

inauspicious; baleful, ill-omened, disastrous.

"He looked upon every instance of bad luck as a **sinistrous** omen of what was awaiting him in the future."

Related word: **sinistrously** (SIN-ə-strəs-lee) *adverb*.

Sisyphean (SIS-ə-FEE-ən)

From the name **Sisyphus** (SIS-ə-fəs), in transliterated Greek written *Sisypheios*, a minor figure in Greek legend who was condemned for his trickery and punished by the gods by being forced forever to roll a boulder uphill.

Unfortunately for him, each time he got near the top the boulder would slip from his grasp and roll all the way downhill. This gave us the phrases **Sisyphean task, Sisyphean labor,** and the rest for an "impossibly hard, never-ending job."

of a task: endless and unavailing.

"Among the many **Sisyphean** odd jobs he was told to do was that of daily scrubbing the many lavatories and their toilets, which were used and abused all day and night."

slatternly (SLAT-ərn-lee)

An ugly English word from English **slattern,** meaning "slut, harlot"; perhaps from **slatter,** an archaic verb meaning "to spill or splash."

of persons: slovenly, untidy; having such ways.

"When she left her job, she began to neglect her appearance and soon became **slatternly**."

Related words: **slatternly** (SLAT-ərn-lee) *adverb*; **slattern** (SLAT-ərn) *noun*.

sloe-eyed (SLOH-ID)

From German *Schlehe*, meaning "sloe; wild plum," + English **-eyed**.

The sloe is *Prunus spinosa*, a name that suggests thorny or prickly fruit, and anyone who has been privy to a shot of **sloe gin** knows its very taste is also thorny or prickly, if that can be imagined. At any rate, we owe thanks to the unrecorded originator of the famous Ramos Gin Fizz, a native New Orleans concoction delicious to the taste, which lives on to this day to remind us that in the right quantity the thorniest addition to any substance can result in a thing of beauty.

dark-eyed; having very dark eyes naturally or through artifice.

> "Whenever the **sloe-eyed** girl known as Tangerine entered any nightclub in the French Quarter, the music stopped at once, and the band went immediately into her theme song."

Related word: **sloe** (sloh) *noun*.

sluggardly (SLUG-ərd-lee)

From the English noun **sluggard**, from **slug**, an archaic verb meaning "to be sluggish"; from Middle English *slogarde*, a noun meaning "sluggardly or slothful person." The adjective is also given as **sluggard** (SLUG-ərd).

slothful; lazy, indolent.

> "There was no question that a **sluggardly** person unused to the rapid-fire questions facing him every day would not last very long in the new job."

Related words: **sluggard** (SLUG-ərd) *noun* and *adjective*; **sluggardliness** (SLUG-ərd-lee-nis) *noun*.

See also **cunctative**.

snafu (sna-FOO)

From American World War II military slang, acronym for "situation normal: all fucked up," expressing the dogged resignation of infantrymen who are accustomed to periods of waiting and to uncomfortable and generally disagreeable conditions induced by uncaring and inexperienced second lieutenants who lack even perfunctory knowledge of combat.

Also given as "situation normal: all fouled up" when explaining the vicissitudes of warfare to innocent civilians and to baby-faced lieutenants.

Our rich language also attempted to establish **fubar** (FOO-bar) to convey the same meaning given by **snafu**, suggesting fucked up beyond all recognition, with the bowdlerized fouled up also provided as more suitable than fucked up for a younger audience. But this fanciful acronym seems to have disappeared.

chaotic, confused, muddled.

> "Anyone who knows the fellow and his ways will surely understand why everything he does is usually **snafu**."

snide (snīd)
> Of uncertain origin.

> 1. slyly derogatory.

> "Larry was a **snide** smart aleck who used public criticism of his students to show off his superiority."

> 2. insinuating, sneering.

> "The agony of sitting through one hour of the young professor's **snide** evaluations of our term papers would readily show why we object to his gaining tenure."

> Related word: **snideness** (SNĪD-nis) *noun.*

soigné (swahn-YAY)
> From the French past participle of the infinitive *soigner*, meaning "to take care of"; from *soin*, meaning "a care." Also given in the feminine form as **soignée**.

> well groomed; carefully prepared, designed, or dressed; sophisticated.

> "The aging actress was still perfectly **soignée** when she appeared in public even though she had not made a movie in years."

solicitous (sə-LIS-i-təs)
> From Latin *sollicitus*, meaning "anxious, troubled"; from infinitive *sollicitare*, meaning "to agitate, excite."

> eager; anxious and concerned about; taking utmost heed or care.

> "He was always **solicitous** of his mother's well-being even when there were others to look after her."

> Related words: **solicit** (sə-LIS-it) *verb*; **solicitor** (sə-LIS-i-tər), **solicitation** (sə-LIS-i-TAY-shən), **solicitude** (sə-LIS-i-TOOD), and **solicitousness** (sə-LIS-i-təs-nis), *all nouns*; **solicitously** (sə-LIS-i-təs-lee) *adverb.*

somnolent (SOM-nə-lənt)
> From Latin *somnolentus*, from *somnus*, meaning "sleep," + **-ulent**, an English suffix borrowed from Latin suffix *-ulentus* and also meaning "full of."

> Also given as **somnifacient** (SOM-nə-FAY-shənt) and **somniferous** (som-NIF-ər-əs). *See* also **soporiferous**.

> of persons: drowsy, sleepy, heavy with sleep; of conditions or drugs: tending to induce sleep.

"There's nothing like the lapping noise of a gentle oceanfront to induce a much-needed **somnolent** state in overstressed men and women."

Related words: **somnolence** (SOM-nə-ləns) and **somnolency** (SOM-nə-lən-see) *both nouns*; **somnolently** (SOM-nə-lənt-lee) *adverb*.

soporiferous (SOP-ə-RIF-ər-əs)

From Latin *soporifer*, meaning "drowsy; causing sleep." *See also* **somnolent**.

soporific; sleepy, drowsy; inducing sleep.

"His specialty was **soporiferous** explanation of phenomena no one cared about or listened to."

Related words: **soporiferously** (SOP-ə-RIF-ər-əs-lee) *adverb*; **soporiferousness** (SOP-ə-RIF-ər-əs-nis) *noun*.

specious (SPEE-shəs)

From Latin *speciosus*, meaning "showy, beautiful; fair."

superficially pleasing; intended to make a favorable impression though lacking real merit.

"We had become accustomed to his **specious** arguments and regarded his promotion to a high position with the greatest skepticism."

Related words: **speciously** (SPEE-shəs-lee) *adverb*; **speciosity** (SPEE-shee-OS-i-tee) and **speciousness** (SPEE-shəs-nis) *both nouns*.

splenetic (spli-NET-ik)

From Late Latin *spleneticus*, from *splen*, meaning the noun "spleen," the organ of the body that old-time physicians used to blame for all who showed signs of peevishness or irritability.

Also given as **splenetical** (spli-NET-i-kəl) and as **splenic** (SPLEE-nik).

Whereas modern physicians identify the psyche—wherever that is—as the source of some persons' physical ailments, it earlier was the custom to blame a specific bodily organ or a misfunctioning thereof for any mystifying symptom, thus enriching our language—**splenetic**, an adjective made from "spleen," is a linguistic hangover of this tendency.

irascible; testy, irritable, spiteful.

"We had to be careful in their house not to irritate their **splenetic** grandfather."

Related word: **splenetically** (spli-NET-i-kə-lee) *adverb.*

spumescent (spyoo-MES-ənt)
From English **spume**, from Latin *spuma*, meaning "foam, froth," + *-escent*, an adjectival suffix meaning "becoming."

foamlike, frothy; foamy.

"The motorboat sped by, leaving a **spumescent** trail hundreds of feet long and rocking all the little boats in its wake."

Related word: **spumescence** (spyoo-MES-əns) *noun.*

spurious (SPYUUR-ee-əs)
From Latin *spurius*, meaning "bastard; false."

not genuine; of illegitimate birth, bastard; adulterous.

"Not until he had been on the job for several years did we learn that his credentials were entirely **spurious**."

Related words: **spuriously** (SPYUUR-ee-əs-lee) *adverb*; **spuriousness** (SPYUUR-ee-əs-nis) *noun.*

staid (stayd)
Adjectival use of English **stayed**, past participle of **stay**.

of a person: of grave deportment, settled in character, dignified in conduct.

"Much to Owen's surprise, his **staid** manners appealed to parents but turned off young girls."

Related words: **staidly** (STAYD-lee) *adverb*; **staidness** (STAYD-nis) *noun.*

steatopygic (stee-AT-ə-PĪ-jik)
From Greek prefix *steat*, meaning "fat," + *o*, to make *steato*, a combining form meaning *fat* + *pyge*, meaning "buttocks."

Also given as **steatopygous** (stee-AT-ə-PĪ-gəs).

said especially of women: given to **steatopygia**, excessive development of fat on the buttocks.

"In some cultures a **steatopygic** physique is considered attractive, in others just something to work off at the gym."

Related word: **steatopygia** (stee-AT-ə-PĪ-jee-ə) *noun.*

stentorian (sten-TOR-ee-ən)

From Stentor, the name of a Greek warrior in the Trojan War. According to Homer, "his voice was as powerful as fifty combined voices of other men."

Also given as **stentorious** (sten-TOR-ee-əs).

of the voice or uttered sounds: very loud or powerful.

"The principal's **stentorian** commands needed no microphone to amplify his orders."

Related words: **stentorianly** (sten-TOR-ee-ən-lee) and **stentoriously** (sten-TOR-ee-əs-lee) *both adverbs.*

stertorous (STUR-tər-əs)

From English **stertor,** meaning "a heavy snoring sound," from Latin infinitive *stertere,* meaning "to snore."

sounding like breathing in the manner of snoring; characterized by snoring.

"His **stertorous** breathing indicated that he was finally asleep, but the snoring was keeping me awake."

Related words: **stertorously** (STUR-tər-əs-lee) *adverb;* **stertorousness** (STUR-tər-əs-nis) *noun.*

straitlaced (STRAYT-LAYST)

From Middle English *streit,* from Latin *strictus,* past participle of infinitive *stringere,* meaning "to bind," + *laced,* past participle of infinitive *laqueare,* meaning "to enclose in a noose"; from *laqueus,* meaning "a noose, snare, halter, trap."

of persons: prudish, puritanical, excessively strict in conduct or morality. Mistakenly spelled **straightlaced.**

"Most of my friends are careful in their customs and behavior, but not to the point of being **straitlaced.**"

Related words: **straitlacedly** (STRAYT-LAY-sid-lee) *adverb;* **straitlacedness** (STRAYT-LAY-sid-nis) *noun.*

stramineous (strə-MIN-ee-əs)

From Latin *stramineus,* meaning "of straw"; from *stramen* or *stramentum,* meaning "straw, litter," which is straw, hay, or the like used as bedding for animals.

resembling straw; straw colored.

"Rebecca, out in the sun all summer, had seen her hair turn **stramineous.**"

strepitous (STREP-i-təs)

From Latin *strepitus*, meaning "noise, clatter"; from *strepere*, infinitive meaning "to make a noise," and Italian *strepitoso*, meaning "noisy," generally a musical term.

Also given as **strepitant** (STREP-i-tənt).

noisy, boisterous; accompanied by much noise.

"I found the sound track so **strepitous** that I could not follow the dialogue."

stridulous (STRIJ-ə-ləs)

From Latin *stridulus*, meaning "creaking, hissing, whistling"; from infinitive *stridere*, meaning "to creak, hiss, shriek, whistle."

Also given as **stridulant** (STRIJ-ə-lənt).

emitting or producing a shrill grating sound; of a voice or sound: harsh, shrill, grating.

"The piercing screaming of her **stridulous** children gave me a headache."

Related words: **stridulously** (STRIJ-ə-ləs-lee) *adverb*; **stridulousness** (STRIJ-ə-ləs-nis) *noun*.

stupefacient (STOO-pə-FAY-shənt)

From Latin *stupefaciens*, present participle of infinitive *stupefacere*, meaning "to stun, astound."

Also given as **stupefactive** (STOO-pə-FAK-tiv).

stupefying; producing stupor.

"By the time he had sipped enough of the liquor to realize it was **stupefacient**, he knew he had already begun to lapse into happy unconsciousness."

Related words: **stupefyingly** (STOO-pə-FT-ing-lee) *adverb*; **stupefaction** (STOO-pə-FAK-shən), **stupefiedness** (STOO-pə-FTD-nis), and **stupefier** (STOO-pə-FT-ər), *all nouns*; **stupefy** (STOO-pə-FT) *verb*.

subfuscous (sub-FUS-kəs)

From Latin *subfuscus*, from prefix *sub-*, meaning "nearly," + *fuscus*, meaning "dark, swarthy."

Also given as slang **subfusc** (sub-FUSK).

of dusky, somber, or dull hue; dingy, drab.

"She had a sunny, optimistic disposition, so I was surprised when I saw her painting to discover that she used a **subfuscous** palette."

succedent (sək-SEED-nt)

From Latin *succedens,* present participle of infinitive *succedere,* meaning "to succeed."

Also given as **succeeding** (sək-SEE-ding).

subsequent; following, succeeding.

"Little is known of the formal proceedings of the society in its first years, but **succedent** generations have left detailed, informative accounts of the monthly meetings."

Related words: **succeed** (sək-SEED) *verb;* **succeedingly** (sək-SEED-ing-lee) *adverb;* **succeedable** (sək-SEED-ə-bəl) *adjective;* **succeeder** (sək-SEED-ər) *noun.*

succinct (sək-SINGKT)

From Latin *succinctus,* past participle of infinitive *succingere,* from *sub-,* meaning "under," + *cingere,* meaning "to gird."

We can think of *succingere,* then, as "to prepare for action: gird up, tuck up, equip, arm." And we can understand how all these latter definitions can be part of preparing for action.

of a story: brief and concise; compressed, expressed in few words.

"Professor Goodman made much of the importance of offering **succinct** verbal pictures in order to achieve realistic, fast-moving fiction."

Related words: **succinctly** (sək-SINGKT-lee) *adverb;* **succinctness** (sək-SINGKT-nis) *noun.*

sudorific (soo-də-RIF-ik)

From Latin *sudorificus,* from *sudor,* meaning "sweat, perspiration; hard work, exertion"; from infinitive *sudare,* meaning "to sweat."

Also given as **sudoriferous** (soo-də-RIF-ər-əs) and **sudoriparous** (soo-də-RIP-ər-əs).

diaphoretic; perspiratory; promoting or causing perspiration.

"Eating has a **sudorific** effect on Andy Sipowicz, which he feels impelled to explain to his dates."

Related word: **sudoriferousness** (soo-də-RIF-ər-əs-nis) *noun.*

superannuated (soo-pər-AN-yoo-AY-tid)

From Medieval Latin *superannatus*, said of cattle and meaning "over a year old," from *super* "beyond" + *annum* "a year."

1. of persons: disqualified or incapacitated by age or infirmities.

   "Only when it happens to you can you begin to understand what it means to be told you are **superannuated** and must, therefore, accept the idea there is no place for you anymore in the organization to which you have given most of your life."

2. of things or abstractions: antiquated, worn out, obsolete.

   "Most of my own ideas have been discarded as **superannuated** even though I believe they are as good as anything around today."

   Related words: **superannuate** (soo-pər-AN-yoo-AYT) *verb*; **superannuation** (soo-pər-AN-yoo-AY-shən) *noun*.

supercilious (soo-pər-SIL-ee-əs)

From Latin *superciliosus*, from *supercilium*, meaning "eyebrow," from *super-*, a prefix meaning "above" + *cilium*, meaning "eyelid."

The most interesting aspect of *supercilium* is that it also means "arrogance." So now we understand an important rôle of the eyebrow.

haughtily contemptuous in character or behavior; marked by an air of contemptuous superiority or disdain; dictatorial, arbitrary, overbearing.

   "His **supercilious** arrogance is deflated only when he is discovered to have made a flagrant error."

   Related words: **superciliously** (soo-pər-SIL-ee-əs-lee) *adverb*; **superciliary** (soo-pər-SIL-ee-ER-ee) *adjective*; **superciliousness** (soo-pər-SIL-ee-əs-nis) *noun*.

supine (soo-PĪN)

From Latin *supinus*, meaning "lying on one's back faceup" and "inactive."

These definitions lent the imprimatur of Roman notions of character to our stern schoolmasters of generations past who endlessly preached the need for industrious scholars to sit straight up in their seats if they wanted ever to achieve anything worthwhile in life.

1. lying on the back; face or front upward.

   "He understood that landing **supine** after an enemy bomb had exploded near him had kept his nose above the sea of mud around him and made it possible for him to breathe until he was rescued by men in his squad."

2. morally or mentally inactive; inert, indolent.

"Fortunately, Edmund soon realized he had been leading a **supine** life unsuitable for a person of his great talent and mental ability."

Related words: **supinely** (soo-PĪN-lee) *adverb*; **supineness** (soo-PĪN-nis) *noun.*

susurrant (suu-SUR-ənt)

From Latin *susurrans*, present participle of infinitive *susurrare*, meaning "to murmur, buzz, whisper."

The adjective **susurrous** (suu-SUR-əs) is also heard.

of the nature of a whisper; full of whispering or murmuring sounds.

"The **susurrant** wind in the trees had the effect of lulling me to sleep."

Related words: **susurration** (soo-sə-RAY-shən) and **susurrus** (suu-SUR-əs) *both nouns.*

synergetic (SIN-ər-JET-ik)

From Greek *synergetikós*, from prefix *syn-*, meaning "together," + *ergetikos*, a form of the infinitive *ergein*, meaning "to be active."

cooperative; working together.

"One of his goals was to exploit the full benefits of **synergetic** activity in his department so that each element would profit from cooperation with other elements."

Related words: **synergism** (SIN-ər-JIZ-əm) and **synergy** (SIN-ər-jee) *both nouns*; **synergistic** (SIN-ər-JIS-tik) and **synergic** (si-NUR-jik) *both adjectives*; **synergistically** (SIN-ər-JIS-tik-kə-lee) *adverb.*

T

tabescent (tə-BES-ənt)

From Latin *tabescens*, present participle of *tabescere*, meaning "beginning to waste away"; from infinitive *tabere*, meaning "to waste away."

Also given as **tabetic** (tə-BET-ik).

becoming emaciated; wasting away.

"The **tabescent** model's appearance led us to wonder whether she would survive the demands of our autumn schedule."

Related words: **tabes** (TAY-beez) and **tabescence** (tə-BES-əns) *both nouns.*

tacit (TAS-it)

From Latin *tacitus*, meaning "silent," past participle of infinitive *tacere*, meaning "to be silent." *See also* **taciturn**.

implicit, understood; unspoken, unvoiced; saying nothing, still, silent.

"I thought we had your **tacit** approval of the entire scheme when you said there was no need for a written agreement."

Related words: **tacitly** (TAS-it-lee) *adverb;* **tacitness** (TAS-it-nis) *noun.*

taciturn (TAS-i-TURN)

From Latin *taciturnus*, meaning "quiet, silent."

See also **tacit.**

of few words, saying little; characterized by disinclination to conversation; uncommunicative.

"Imagine my dismay when I found I was seated between two **taciturn** bankers who would never say a word."

Related words: **taciturnly** (TAS-i-TURN-lee) *adverb*; **taciturnity** (TAS-i-TUR-ni-tee) *noun*.

tactless (TAKT-lis)

From English **tact,** meaning "sensitivity," + **-less,** a suffix meaning "without."

showing no tact; offendingly blunt.

"He said his shin was raw after a dinner during which he was kicked by his wife under the table every time he let fly with one of his **tactless** remarks."

Related words: **tactlessly** (TAKT-lis-lee) *adverb*; **tactlessness** (TAKT-lis-nis) *noun*.

tangential (tan-JEN-shəl)

From English **tangent,** meaning "slightly connected," + **-ial,** an adjectival suffix meaning "of the type of."

digressive; divergent; merely touching a subject or matter.

"Much of what he said to us was at best only **tangential** to our true concerns and not worth the time and attention we were obliged to give it."

Related words: **tangentially** (tan-JEN-shə-lee) *adverb*; **tangentiality** (tan-JEN-shee-AL-i-tee) *noun*.

tarty (TAHR-tee)

From English noun **tart,** meaning "a prostitute or promiscuous woman or girl," + **-y,** an adjectival suffix meaning "inclined to."

cheap; suggestive of a woman of low moral character.

"When he brought a **tarty** looking woman to a family dinner, we concluded he was either deliberately trying to offend us or had taken leave of his senses."

Related word: **tart** (tahrt) *noun*.

temerarious (TEM-ə-RAIR-ee-əs)

From Latin *temerarius,* meaning "accidental, rash, thoughtless"; from *temere,* an adverb meaning "by chance, at random; rashly, thoughtlessly"; from the noun *temeritas,* meaning "chance, rashness, thoughtlessness."

rash; reckless, heedless; unreasonably adventurous.

"The inexperienced young man's **temerarious** venture into the world of finance was immediately seen as an ill-advised disaster."

Related words: **temerariously** (TEM-ə-RAIR-ee-əs-lee) *adverb*; **temerariousness** (TEM-ə-RAIR-ee-əs-nis) and **temerity** (tə-MER-i-tee) *both nouns.*

tendentious (ten-DEN-shəs)

From Medieval Latin *tendentia*, meaning "tendency," + *-ous*, an adjectival suffix meaning "possessing."

showing or having a definite bias, purpose, or tendency.

"The first plan was never seriously considered because the author's motivation was so obviously **tendentious**."

Related words: **tendency** (TEN-dən-see) and **tendentiousness** (ten-DEN-shəs-nis) *both nouns*; **tendentiously** (ten-DEN-shəs-lee) *adverb.*

tenebrous (TEN-ə-brəs)

From Latin *tenebrosus*, meaning "dark, gloomy"; from *tenebrae*, meaning "darkness, night; unconsciousnees, death, blindness."

Also given as **tenebrious** (tə-NEB-ree-əs), meaning "dark, gloomy," and **tenebrific** (TEN-ə-BRIF-ik), meaning "producing darkness."

gloomy; dark, obscure.

"The campers hoped that the pale dawn light would bring to a happy conclusion their **tenebrous** forebodings."

tenuous (TEN-yuu-əs)

From Latin *tenuis*, meaning "thin."

of slight significance; having little substance or validity; thin in form or consistency.

"The **tenuous** defense the attorney offered surprised all of us at the time but finally was shown to have much more substance than we had thought."

Related words: **tenuity** (tə-NOO-i-tee) and **tenuousness** (TEN-yoo-əs-nis) *both nouns*; **tenuously** (TEN-yoo-əs-lee) *adverb.*

tepid (TEP-id)

From Latin *tepidus*, meaning "warm, lukewarm," from infinitive *tepere*, meaning "to be lukewarm."

Some insight is provided into the figurative meaning of **tepid** by a secondary meaning of the Latin verb *tepere*, "to be in love." An extraordinary linguistic insight of Romans, who clearly suggested there were degrees of romantic interest.

lukewarm; moderately warm; unenthusiastic; lacking force.

> "The **tepid** reviews her book began to receive were disappointing and dispiriting."

Related words: **tepidly** (TEP-id-lee) *adverb*; **tepidity** (te-PID-i-tee) and **tepidness** (TEP-id-nis) *both nouns*.

testate (TES-tayt)

From Latin *testatus*, past participle of infinitive *testari*, meaning "to bear witness; to make a will"; from the noun *testis*, "a witness."

But, of course, the English **testis** (TES-tis) also means "testicle," in Latin usually given as *testiculus*. Until the present, no one has managed to make the act of swearing an oath more convincing than the way the Romans did it, finding the grabbing of one's own genitals infinitely more demonstrative than holding one's right hand upward while touching a Bible with the left. Yet we immmediately notice the linguistic similarity between **testament** and **testicle**— both eventually from *testari*, as shown above.

Testate is one of those positive words that are made negative by adding the prefix **in-**, meaning "not." Yet we are more accustomed to the orneriness of dying Americans who willingly go to their great reward **intestate** (in-TES-tayt) than we are to the somewhat lesser number who willfully prefer to be **testate**. (All puns here are intentional.)

of a person: someone who has left a valid will at death.

> "It makes life much easier for heirs who find out that persons they mourn have died **testate** rather than intestate."

Related words: **testacy** (TES-tə-see) *noun*; **testamentary** (TES-tə-MEN-tə-ree) *adjective*; **testator** (TES-tay-tər) and **testatrix** (te-STAY-triks) *both nouns*.

testis. *See* testate.

thaumaturgic (THAW-mə-TUR-jik)

From Greek *thaumatourgós*, from *thaumato-*, meaning "miracle, wonder," + *-ourgos*, meaning "work," + *-ic*, an adjectival suffix meaning "having the characteristic of."

Also given as **thaumaturgical** (THAW-mə-TUR-ji-kəl).

wonder-working; with the power of performing miracles or marvels.

> "Who does not wistfully long to recapture an innocent belief in such **thaumaturgic** institutions as a magician's tricks, Santa Claus, and the tooth fairy?"

Related words: **thaumaturge** (THAW-mə-TURJ) and **thaumaturgy** (THAW-mə-TUR-jee) *both nouns.*

thersitical (thər-SIT-i-kəl)

In Greek legend *Thersites* (thər-SĪ-teez) was an unpopular Greek officer at the siege of Troy—deformed, abusive, reviling, scurrilous, and given to railing at his chiefs.

And how did things turn out for Thersites? Achilles, with but a single punch, knocked him down and permanently out.

scurrilous; foul-mouthed, reviling.

"All I remember about the company first sergeant is that he never missed a chance to be vicious and **thersitical**."

thrasonical (thray-SAHN-i-kəl)

From the name of the braggart Thraso in the play *Eunuchus* by the Roman playwright Terence, the Latin *Eunuchus* in the title, of course, meaning "a eunuch."

vainglorious; bragging, boastful.

"He thought he was impressing her with accounts of his accomplishments, but actually she was repelled by his **thrasonical** rambling."

timorous (TIM-ər-əs)

From Latin *timor*, meaning "fear, alarm; a terror," + *-osus*, akin to English **-ous**, an adjectival suffix meaning "full of."

fearful; frightened, apprehensive; timid.

"Characteristically, he was so **timorous** that he stayed behind on shore while all the other boys ran recklessly into the rapids and were immediately swept away, never to be heard from again."

Related words: **timorously** (TIM-ər-əs-lee) *adverb*; **timorousness** (TIM-ər-əs-nis) *noun.*

tintinnabular (TIN-ti-NAB-yə-lər)

From Latin *tintinnabulum*, meaning "a small tinkling bell"; from infinitive *tintinare*, meaning "to ring."

Also given as **tintinabulary** (TIN-ti-NAB-yə-LER-ee) and as **tintinnabulous** (TIN-ti-NAB-yə-ləs).

pertaining to bells or bell ringing.

"The **tintinnabular** sound of the familiar church bells never fails to thrill me."

Related word: **tintinnabulation** (TIN-ti-NAB-yə-LAY-shən) *noun.*

titian (TISH-ən)

From the name Titian (Tiziano Vecellio), a great Italian artist who died in 1576, leaving several paintings in which **titian**-color hair was painted.

having reddish brown (titian) hair, also expressed as bright golden auburn hair.

"Hazel's **titian** hair was burnished in the sunlight, which brought out all its red and gold."

tonsorial (ton-SOR-ee-əl)

From Latin *tonsorius*, meaning "for shaving"; from infinitive *tondere*, meaning "to shave."

often used humorously: pertaining to a barber or his work of trimming hair.

"His business cards identified him as "Al, Your Friendly **Tonsorial** Artist.""

toothsome (TOOTH-səm)

From English **tooth,** which everybody knows, + **-some,** an adjectival suffix; hence a word meaning "palatable" as well as "sexually enticing or alluring."

1. savory, appetizing; attractive to the palate.

"To top off an evening of fine dining, our hostess served us a **toothsome** collection of five-flavored ice creams atop a sponge cake, all of which she had prepared from start to finish."

2. voluptuous; sexually alluring.

"Little did she know her husband had arranged for us to be escorted that evening by three **toothsome** Hollywood starlets."

Related words: **toothsomely** (TOOTH-səm-lee) *adverb;* **toothsomeness** (TOOTH-səm-nis) *noun.*

torpid (TOR-pid)

From Latin *torpidus*, meaning "numb, benumbed," from infinitive *torpere*, meaning "to be stiff or numb; to be stupefied."

Also given as **torporific** (TOR-pə-RIF-ik).

dormant, benumbed; slow, sluggish; apathetic, stupefied.

"A heavy dinner left us **torpid,** too dull to appreciate the fine play we were seeing."

Related words: **torpidly** (TOR-pid-lee) *adverb;* **torpor** (TOR-pər), **torpidity** (tor-PID-i-tee), and **torpidness** (TOR-pid-nis) *all nouns.*

tortuous (TOR-choo-əs)

From Latin *tortuosus,* meaning "winding; complicated."

See also the word **torturous** (TOR-chər-əs), which follows.

1. twisting, turning; sinuous.

"Fred did not know his passenger was rigid with fear as he maneuvered the **tortuous** hairpin turns of the mountain road."

2. devious; crooked; indirect, circuitous.

"The last advice he was given was to be on his guard when dealing with her **tortuous** schemes."

Related words: **tortuously** (TOR-choo-əs-lee) *adverb;* **tortuousness** (TOR-choo-əs-nis) *noun.*

torturous (TOR-chər-əs)

From Late Latin *tortura,* meaning "torture."

Remember that a **tortuous** presentation is full of twists and turns, but **torturous** treatment involves physical and emotional suffering and can make you sorry you ever were born.

excruciating; involving or causing suffering or torture.

"Interrogations in prison camps are typically long and **torturous,** almost inevitably resulting in false confessions."

Related words: **torture** (TOR-chər) *verb* and *noun;* **torturously** (TOR-chər-əs-lee) *adverb.*

tramontane (trə-MON-tayn)

From Latin *transmontanus,* literally meaning "beyond the mountains," also given as **transmontane** (trans-mon-TAYN), and just another way of indicating the narrowness of people who live in big cities.

Among the Romans this was a way of saying "on the other side of the Alps," which meant a place so foreign and obscure that when you got there you were nowhere. Sort of like North Dakota.

Little did the Romans know that at the same time the Swiss, the actual **tramontane** people they derogated, also managed to think of the Romans, their big city cousins, as being the people "on the other side of the Alps."

foreign, barbarous; being from the boondocks, the other side of the mountains.

"Never did most of the people speak out against the **tramontane** interlopers until they realized that native citizens constituted less than half the country's population."

transmontane. *See* **tramontane.**

traumatic (trə-MAT-ik)

From Greek *traumatikós*, meaning "pertaining to wounds."

caused by a wound or an emotional shock; psychologically painful.

"Separation of children from their parents had an even more **traumatic** effect than the bombings themselves."

Related words: **traumatically** (trə-MAT-i-kə-lee) *adverb*; **trauma** (TROW-mə) and **traumatology** (TROW-mə-TOL-ə-jee) *both nouns*; **traumatize** (TROW-mə-TIZ) *verb*.

tremulous (TREM-yə-ləs)

From Latin *tremulus*, an adjective meaning "trembling, shivering"; from infinitive *tremere*, meaning "to tremble, to shake."

Also given as **tremulant** (TREM-yə-lənt).

1. of persons: affected by trembling or quivering from weakness or from fear or nervous agitation.

"By the time David had recovered his voice, it was so **tremulous** that few of us were able to understand what he was trying to say."

2. of things or handwriting: characterized by trembling or vibration; vibratory, easily caused to tremble.

"His handwriting had become so **tremulous** after his illness that it was barely legible."

Related words: **tremulously** (TREM-yə-ləs-lee) *adverb*; **tremorous** (TREM-ər-əs) *adjective*; **tremulousness** (TREM-yə-ləs-nis) and **tremor** (TREM-ər) *both nouns*.

trenchant (TREN-chənt)

From Old French *trenchant*, present participle of infinitive *trenchier*, meaning "to cut."

incisive, vigorous and clear; effective, energetic; sharply defined.

"The columnist's **trenchant** wit may have caused a few to wince as they read, but no reader could claim that any of the columns she wrote were actually unfair."

Related words: **trench** (trench) *verb;* **trenchantly** (TREN-chənt-lee) adverb; **trenchancy** (TREN-chən-see) *noun.*

trepid (TREP-id)

From Latin *trepidus,* meaning "scared, alarmed; alarming, perilous."

Trepid is a word we may not know until we think for a moment of its better-known cousin **intrepid,** meaning "dauntless, fearless." No one ever named a battleship *The Trepid,* did they?

Also given as **trepidant** (TREP-i-dənt), from the present participle of the infinitive *trepidare,* meaning "to be agitated, bustle about."

apprehensive; fearful, trembling from fear.

"The **trepid** little boy took the hand of the equally fearful young girl as they stepped onto the dance floor for their first dancing lesson."

Related word: **trepidation** (TREP-i-DAY-shən) *noun.*

troglodytic (TROG-lə-DIT-ik)

From Latin *troglodyta,* from Greek *troglodytes,* meaning "cave dweller"; literally, "one who crawls into holes."

The ancient Greeks gave the name **troglodytes** (TROG-lə-DĪTS) to uncivilized people who lived in caves or holes in the ground. Best known among them were said to be the subterranean types who lived in Ethiopia.

Also given as **troglodytical** (TROG-lə-DIT-i-kəl).

1. cave dwelling; having the habits of reclusive persons living in holes in the ground.

"Patient digging by dozens of graduate students enabled paleontologists to publish revealing accounts of the **troglodytic** lives of prehistoric humankind."

2. hermitic; withdrawn from the affairs of the world.

"Once the neighbor's children had left home and never returned, she and her husband withdrew into **troglodytic** existences, leaving their house only to shop for necessities."

Related words: **troglobiont** (TROG-lə-BĪ-ənt), **troglobite** (TROG-lə-BĪT), and **troglodytism** (TROG-lə-dī-TIZ-əm) *all nouns.*

truculent (TRUK-yə-lənt)

From Latin *truculentus,* meaning "ferocious, grim, wild"; from *trux,* meaning "savage, fierce."

1. vitriolic; scathing, savage; brutally harsh.

"Almost every word in his **truculent** paragraphs of criticism seems to have been written with a pen dipped in venom."

2. barbarous; aggressively hostile; fierce, cruel.

"The **truculent** enemy left needlessly burned villages and savagely slain victims in its wake."

Related words: **truculence** (TRUK-yə-ləns) and **truculency** (TRUK-yə-lən-see) *both nouns*; **truculently** (TRUK-yə-lənt-lee) *adverb.*

tumid (TOO-mid)

From Latin *tumidus*, meaning "swollen, swelling"; from infinitive *tumere*, meaning "to swell."

It is important to note that *tumidus* also has the meanings of "bombastic" and "excited and enraged."

1. of a body part: swollen, bulging.

"When the doctor saw my **tumid** foot, which could no longer fit into my shoe, he immediately recognized a case of gout."

2. of pompous language: turgid; inflated, bombastic.

"Her writing was **tumid** and pretentious rather than incisive, as she had intended."

Related words: **tumidly** (TOO-mid-lee) *adverb*; **tumidity** (too-MID-i-tee) and **tumidness** (TOO-mid-nis) *noun.*

turgescent (tur-JES-ənt)

From Latin *turgescens*, present participle of infinitive *turgescere*, meaning "to swell up, begin to swell."

A note on mental health: the Latin verb is also translated as "to become enraged." Be careful.

becoming swollen; swelling, growing bigger.

"In time her **turgescent** breasts will undoubtedly prove more than adequate for feeding the new infant."

See also **turgid.**

Related words: **turgor** (TUR-gər), **turgescence** (tur-JES-əns), and **turgescency** (tur-JES-ən-see) *all nouns.*

turgid (TUR-jid)

From Latin *turgidus*, meaning "swollen or distended; bombastic";

from infinitive *turgere,* meaning "to swell, be swollen." The verb *turgere* may also be translated as "to be bombastic."

See also **tumid.**

1. distended; swollen, puffed out.

"Especially because early fighters' fists were not padded with gloves, it was not uncommon after a bout to be unable to see eyes in the **turgid** faces of the competitors."

2. of language: tumid; inflated, grandiloquent, bombastic.

"Jack found it next to impossible to write simply and clearly, instead preferring **turgid** prose."

Related words: **turgidity** (tur-JID-i-tee) and **turgidness** (TUR-jid-nis) *both nouns;* **turgidly** (TUR-jid-lee) *adverb.*

U

ubiquitous (yoo-BIK-wi-təs)

From Neo-Latin *ubiquitarius,* meaning "everywhere at once"; in English given formerly as *ubiquitary;* from Latin adverb *ubique,* meaning "everywhere."

omnipresent; present or appearing everywhere; everywhere at the same time.

"Jack on his first trip to Paris found it true that everywhere he went he could find one of the **ubiquitous** little cafés he had been told to expect."

Related words: **ubiquity** (yoo-BIK-wi-tee) and **ubiquitousness** (yoo-BIK-wi-təs-nis) *both nouns;* **ubiquitously** (yoo-BIK-wi-təs-lee) *adverb.*

ufological (YOO-fə-LOJ-i-kəl)

From English **u**nidentified **f**lying **o**bject + **-logy,** combining form meaning "study of."

of or pertaining to the study of so-called unidentified flying objects.

"Ramon was spending all his time reading what purported to be authentic **ufological** reports of sightings of strange celestial phenomena."

Related words: **ufology** (yoo-FOL-ə-jee) and **ufologist** (yoo-FOL-ə-jist) *both nouns.*

uliginous (yoo-LIJ-ə-nəs)

From Latin *uliginosus,* meaning "wet, full of moisture"; from *uligo,* meaning "moisture, marshiness."

Also given as **uliginose** (yoo-LIJ-ə-NOHS).

swampy; slimy; of marshes or water-logged places.

"An unusually long rainy season made the region especially **uliginous** that year."

ulotrichous (yoo-LOT-ri-kəs)

From Greek *oulótrichos*, meaning "curly haired"; from *oûlos*, "crisp, curly," + *-trichos*, a combining form meaning "haired," from *thrix*, meaning "hair."

of a group of people said to have what was called woolly hair.

"Europeans exploring continents away from home mistakenly reported they had discovered new species of mankind when they observed **ulotrichous** men and women for the first time."

Related word: **ulotrichy** (yoo-LOT-ri-kee) *noun.*

ululant (UL-yə-lənt)

From Latin *ululans*, present participle of infinitive *ululare*, meaning "to shriek, howl"; perhaps of imitative origin.

having the character of ululation; howling, wailing.

"The **ululant** wolves kept them awake until daybreak, when almost on signal the beasts suddenly stopped their yowling."

Related words: **ululate** (UL-yə-LAYT) *verb*; **ululation** (UL-yə-LAY-shən) *noun.*

umbrageous (um-BRAY-jəs)

From English **umbrage**, meaning "shadowy appearance; offense, annoyance"; from Latin *umbra*, meaning "shade, shadow; ghost."

See also **umbriferous.**

1. shady; forming or affording shade; abounding in shade.

"Our architect told us that in a few years the driveway to our house would be **umbrageous** unless we controlled the growth of our trees."

2. of persons: jealous, suspicious; inclined or apt to take offense.

"In the little town the only persons I found to be **umbrageous** were the old-timers, perhaps because they were afraid of the other changes that newcomers were bringing."

Related words: **umbrageously** (um-BRAY-jəs-lee) *adverb*; **umbrageousness** (um-BRAY-jəs-nis) and **umbrage** (UM-brij) *both nouns.*

umbriferous (um-BRIF-ər-əs)

From Latin *umbrifer*, meaning "shady, shade bringing."

umbrageous; affording shade.

"The old elm provided an **umbriferous** place in which to rest after hiking in the noonday sun."

Related words: **umbriferously** (um-BRIF-ər-əs-lee) *adverb*; **umbriferousness** (um-BRIF-ər-əs-nis) *noun*.

unambiguous (UN-am-BIG-yoo-əs). *See* **unequivocal.**

unconscionable (un-KON-shə-nə-bəl)

From English **un-,** meaning "not," + **conscience,** meaning "the sense of what is right and what is wrong."

1. unscrupulous; not guided by conscience; free from anxiety.

"They accused me of being an **unconscionable** old thief who would steal from his own grandmother if he could get away with it."

2. extortionate; outrageous, excessive.

"That hardware store charges **unconscionable** prices for its merchandise and manages to get away with the practice because it is the only store of its type for miles around."

Related words: **unconscionably** (un-KON-shə-nə-blee) *adverb*; **unconscionableness** (un-KON-shə-nə-bəl-nis) *noun*.

unctuous (UNGK-choo-əs)

From Medieval Latin *unctuosus,* from Latin *unctus,* meaning "the act of anointing," from infinitive *unguere,* meaning "to anoint, smear, grease."

1. smug; excessively pious; excessively smooth.

"While some were flattered by his obsequious attentions, others thought he was an **unctuous** social climber."

2. oily, greasy.

"The **unctuous** matter that exuded from the infection had so bad an odor that it caused some of the medical students to gag."

Related words: **unction** (UNGK-shən), **unctuousness** (UNGK-choo-əs-nis), and **unctuosity** (UNGK-choo-OS-i-tee) *all nouns*; **unctuously** (UNGK-choo-əs-lee) *adverb*.

undulant (UN-jə-lənt)

From English **undulate,** meaning "to cause to move in waves"; from the Latin adjective *undulatus,* meaning "waved."

undulating; moving in the manner of waves; rising and falling like waves.

"Her **undulant** hula dance was enhanced by the rhythmic movement of her grass skirt."

Related words: **undulate** (UN-jə-LAYT) *verb;* **undulation** (UN-jə-LAY-shən) and **undulator** (UN-jə-LAY-tər) *both nouns;* **undulative** (UN-jə-LAY-tiv) *adjective.*

unequivocal (UN-i-KWIV-ə-kəl)

From English **un-,** meaning "not," + **equivocal,** meaning "ambiguous"; from Late Latin *aequivocus* with the same meaning.

Also given as **unambiguous.**

unambiguous; having only one correct interpretation; absolute, unqualified.

"His **unequivocal** answers to our questions assured us that his research was producing the successful results we all anticipated."

Related words: **unequivocally** (UN-i-KWIV-ə-kə-lee) *adverb;* **unequivocalness** (UN-i-KWIV-ə-kəl-nis) *noun.*

unhinged (un-HINJD)

From English infinitive **unhinge,** meaning "to take a door off its hinges."

of a person: distraught; unsettled, thrown into confusion; of a door: taken off its hinges.

"The bad news the doctor gave proved a terrible shock, and the patient almost became **unhinged.**"

Related words: **unhinge** (un-HINJ) *verb;* **unhingement** (un-HINJ-mənt) *noun.*

unimpeachable (UN-im-PEE-chə-bəl)

From English **un-,** meaning "not," + **impeachable,** meaning "able to call into question."

impeccable; impossible to discredit; above suspicion.

"The defense attorneys knew the case depended on their ability to find a single **unimpeachable** witness whose undisputed testimony would punch holes in the district attorney's case."

Related words: **unimpeachably** (UN-im-PEECH-ə-blee) *adverb;* **unimpeachability** (UN-im-PEECH-ə-BIL-i-tee) and **unimpeachableness** (UN-im-PEECH-ə-bəl-nis) *both nouns.*

unjaundiced (un-JAWN-dist)

From English **un-** + **jaundice,** from Latin *galbinus,* meaning "greenish-yellow."

What is there about green and what is there about yellow that cause us to consider these colors opprobrious? Is this why we formerly held a greenish complexion to be indicative of jealousy and why Shakespeare, in *Othello,* called jealousy a green-eyed monster? And isn't yellow the color indicating jealousy, adultery, and cowardice? So it is far better to be **unjaundiced** than **jaundiced.**

not affected by distorted or prejudiced opinions.

"They thought the expert we hired was too close to the family to be disinterested and asked us to find someone who could look at the evidence with an **unjaundiced** eye."

unmitigated (un-MIT-i-GAY-tid)

From English **mitigate,** from Latin *mitigatus,* past participle of infinitive *mitigare,* meaning "to ripen, soften; calm, pacify."

absolute; not softened or toned down; not softened in regard to intensity or severity.

"In light of his neglect to pack food or clothing for the journey, there was no doubt the situation would turn out to be an **unmitigated** disaster."

unplumbed (un-PLUMD)

From Latin *plumbum,* meaning "lead," + *un-,* meaning "not."

The verb **plumb,** in its various forms, meaning "fathom, completely understand, explore in depth," is often heard, as in "After we had fully **plumbed** his expert knowledge, we had to admit we had known little."

unfathomed, unsounded; not explored in depth, not completely understood.

"She spoke eloquently of what she called the '**unplumbed** childishness of men's imaginations' and the necessity for careful consideration of men's habitual shortcomings."

unrequited (UN-ri-KWĪ-tid)

From English verb **requite,** meaning "make repayment," always useful but now seldom written as an adjective without the negative prefix **un-.**

not reciprocated; not repaid.

"Just about the worst condition known is that of the person smitten with love who one day discovers that his passion is **unrequited**."

untenable (un-TEN-ə-bəl)

From English **tenable;** from Latin infinitive *tenere,* meaning "to hold, keep, possess," + *un-,* meaning "not."

of an argument: incapable of being defended logically.

"He was convinced women could not perform intellectual tasks that men master easily, a position that most intelligent people find **untenable**."

Related words: **untenability** (UN-ten-ə-BIL-i-tee) and **untenable-ness** (un-TEN-ə-bəl-nis) *both nouns.*

unwitting (un-WIT-ing)

From Old English *unwittende,* in English formerly *unweeting,* meaning "unknowing, unconscious."

unheeding; oblivious, unaware; unintentional; having no knowledge of a particular fact or condition.

"He insisted that his most reprehensible remark had been completely **unwitting** and that he would never again say anything like it."

Related words: **unwittingly** (un-WIT-ing-lee) *adverb;* **unwitting-ness** (un-WIT-ing-nis) *noun.*

unwonted (un-WAWN-tid)

From the obsolete English *unwont,* meaning "uncustomary, unwonted."

not customary; infrequent, rare; not usual.

"After an entire day of **unwonted** physical effort, Fred and his wife said they were completely exhausted."

Related words: **unwontedly** (un-WAWN-tid-lee) *adverb;* **unwont-edness** (un-WAWN-tid-nis) *noun.*

urbane (ur-BAYN)

From Latin *urbanus,* meaning "living in a town or city; refined, polite; witty, humorous; impertinent."

suave; having manners that are smooth and polite; showing sophistication in manners and expression.

"Joseph's **urbane** manners, which were an asset for his summer intern's position in a Boston law office, made him seem ridiculous in his job as a construction worker."

Related words: **urbanely** (ur-BAYN-lee) *adverb;* **urbaneness** (ur-BAYN-nis) and **urbanity** (ur-BAN-i-tee) *both nouns.*

uxorial (uk-SOR-ee-əl)
From Latin *uxorius,* meaning "of a wife; fond of his wife."

Also given as **uxorious,** with the same meanings as **uxorial.**

typical of or befitting a wife or wives.

"We all wondered at Gary's strange taste in candidates for marriage partner, his **uxorial** litmus test apparently being whether or not a young woman could cook and keep house."

Related words: **uxor** (UK-sor) and **uxoricide** (uk-SOR-ə-sTD) *both nouns;* **uxorially** (uk-SOR-ee-əl-ee) *adverb.*

uxorious (uk-SOR-ee-əs)
Same origin as **uxorial.**

doting or foolishly fond of one's wife; devotedly attached to her.

"When we were children, we found our father's waiting on our mother hand and foot a bit embarrassing, and as adults we considered this **uxorious** concern something to be hidden from our friends."

Related words: **uxoriously** (uk-SOR-ee-əs-lee), *adverb;* **uxoriousness** (uk-SOR-ee-əs-nis) *noun.*

V

vacuous (VAK-yoo-əs)

From Latin *vacuus*, meaning "empty, void, wanting; vacant."

It is interesting to note that *vacuus* also means "disengaged, at leisure; and worthless." Most engaging of all is the meaning "of a woman, single." So now you know all you want to know of Latin's conceptions of women.

idle, purposeless; empty, lacking ideas, without contents.

"From that moment on, Mother was given to sitting near the front window looking, always looking out at the street with a **vacuous** stare, never really seeing anything."

Related words: **vacuum** (VAK-yoom) and **vacuousness** (VAK-yoo-əs-nis) *both nouns;* **vacuously** (VAK-yoo-əs-lee) *adverb.*

vagarious (və-GAIR-ee-əs)

From English **vagary**, meaning "wandering journey," from Latin infinitive *vagari*, meaning "to wander."

erratic, capricious; characterized by wandering, roaming.

"Mark's **vagarious** forays into the arts were obviously not taken seriously by any of his friends."

Related words: **vagariously** (və-GAIR-ee-əs-lee) *adverb;* **vagary** (və-GAIR-ee *or* VAY-gə-ree) *noun.*

vainglorious (vayn-GLOR-ee-əs)

From Medieval Latin *vana gloria*, meaning "empty ambition, empty boasting."

given to vainglory; characterized by inordinate boasting.

"The official **vainglorious** reports we wrote were intended to give the impression we were winning the war."

Related words: **vaingloriously** (vayn-GLOR-ee-əs-lee) *adverb*; **vainglory** (VAYN-GLOR-ee) and **vaingloriousness** (vain-GLOR-ee-əs-nis) *both nouns.*

valetudinarian (VAL-i-TOOD-n-AIR-ee-ən)

From English **valetudinary**, meaning "chronic invalid"; from Latin *valetudinarius*, meaning "sickly"; from *valetudinarium*, meaning "hospital."

sickly; excessively concerned with the state of one's poor health.

"A **valetudinarian** patient becomes so devoted to discussing his health with anyone who will listen that otherwise sympathetic visitors begin avoiding him."

Related words: **valetudinary** (VAL-i-TOOD-n-ER-ee) and **valetudinarianism** (VAL-i-TOOD-n-AIR-ee-ə-NIZ-əm) *both nouns.*

vapid (VAP-id)

From Latin *vapidus*, meaning "tasteless, insipid"; from *vapor*, meaning "steam; heat."

insipid; having lost sharpness or zest; devoid of animation; dull, tedious.

"Nell's conversation was as **vapid** as her tea, if you can imagine a weak brew steeped in tepid water."

Related words: **vapidly** (VAP-id-lee) *adverb*; **vapidness** (VAP-id-nis) and **vapidity** (və-PID-i-tee) *both nouns.*

varicose (VAR-i-KOHS)

From Latin *varicosus*, meaning "suffering from varicose veins."

swollen; abnormally enlarged.

"She never sat on a beach while dressed for swimming because she was ashamed of revealing her ugly **varicose** veins to her grandchildren."

Related words: **varicosis** (VAR-i-KOH-sis) and **varicosity** (VAR-i-KOS-i-tee) *both nouns.*

variorum (VAIR-ee-OR-əm)

From a shortening of Latin *editio cum notis variorum*, freely translated as "an edition, especially of the complete works of a classical author, containing the notes of various editors or commentators."

containing the notes of various commentators; also, containing various versions of a text by various scholars.

"Arthur had a distinguished career capped by his **variorum** edition of the principal work of America's most illustrious poet."

vatic (VAT-ik)

From Latin *vates*, meaning "poet; prophet."

Also given as **vatical** (VAT-i-kəl).

inspired, prophetic; characteristic of a prophet.

"Much to the surprise of Samantha's ardent admirers, her most important **vatic** pronouncements, so characteristic of her, went unnoticed until long after her death."

Related words: **vaticinal** (və-TIS-ə-nl) *adjective*; **vaticide** (VAT-ə-sīD) and **vaticination** (və-TIS-ə-NAY-shən) *both nouns*; **vaticinate** (və-TIS-ə-NAYT) *verb*.

ventricose (VEN-tri-KOHS)

From Neo-Latin *ventricosus*, from Latin *venter*, meaning "belly."

The adjective **ventricose**, synonymous with "swollen," must not be confused with the archaic adjective **ventose** (VEN-tohs), which means "full of wind, flatulent."

protuberant, bellied; having a large abdomen; swelling out in the middle or the side of an animal's belly.

"The young physician could only guess at the cause of the patient's puzzling **ventricose** symptom, which was giving such discomfort."

Related word: **ventricosity** (VEN-tri-KOS-i-tee) *noun*.

veracious (və-RAY-shəs)

From English **veracity**, from Latin *verax*, meaning "truthful."

Not to be confused with **voracious** (vaw-RAY-shəs), meaning "ravenous." *See also* **veridical**.

truthful; accurate; disposed to express the truth.

"One thing that lawyers have trouble finding is a person who will be perceived by a jury as thoroughly **veracious**."

Related words: **veraciously** (və-RAY-shəs-lee) *adverb*; **veracity** (və-RAS-i-tee) and **veraciousness** (və-RAY-shəs-nis) *both nouns*.

verdurous (VUR-jər-əs)

From English **verdure** (VUR-jər), a noun meaning "greenness, freshness."

The adjective is also given as **verdant** (VUR-dnt).

flourishing rich and green; covered with verdure.

"Earlier, when Tom's aches and pains did not restrict his bending and digging, his **verdurous** gardens were a neighborhood show place."

Related words: **verdantly** (VUR-dnt-lee) *adverb*; **verdancy** (VUR-dn-see) *noun*.

verecund (VER-i-KUND)

From Latin *verecundus*, an adjective meaning "modest, shy, bashful"; from the infinitive *vereri*, meaning "to revere, respect; fear."

Just as Latin words for these expressions of respect appear no longer to be needed, people being what they have become, the English derivative has gone the way of all archaisms. It is included here only because the word is beautiful to the ear and sometimes is found in English novels of centuries past.

modest, bashful; coy, shy.

"I felt sorry for the **verecund** little boy standing outside the headmaster's office, apparently waiting for an interview he rued and had not requested."

Related words: **verecundity** (VER-i-KUND-i-tee) and **verecundness** (VER-i-KUND-nis) *both archaic nouns*.

veridical (və-RID-i-kəl)

From Latin *veridicus*, meaning "truthful"; from *verum*, meaning "truth," + *dicere*, meaning "to speak."

Also given as **veridic** (və-RID-ik) and **veracious,** which see.

veracious; truthful; actual; genuine.

"When I found my superior openly **veridical** in all his opinions, I resolved to complete every word of my report without regard for anyone's feelings."

Related words: **veridically** (və-RID-i-kə-lee) *adverb*; **veridicality** (və-RID-i-KAL-i-tee) *noun*.

vertiginous (vər-TIJ-ə-nəs)

From Latin *vertiginosus*, from *vertigo*, meaning "a turning round, dizziness."

dizzy, giddy; spinning, whirling; unstable, apt to change quickly.

"I immediately regretted taking the pill because for the first time I felt truly **vertiginous** and wondered whether things would ever return to the way they had been."

Related words: **vertigo** (VUR-ti-GOH) and **vertiginousness** (vur-TIJ-ə-nəs-nis) *both nouns;* **vertiginously** (vur-TIJ-i-nəs-lee) *adverb.*

vespertine (VES-pər-tin)

From Latin *vespertinus,* meaning "in the evening" and "western." An indication that the Romans knew their astronomy well, as shown also in two other Latin words, *occidentalis* and *occiduus,* both meaning "western" or "setting."

Also given as **vespertinal** (ves-pər-TĪN-l).

No wonder **vespers** (VES-purz) in Christian customs came to be applied to "evening services."

pertaining to or occurring in the evening.

"It was our custom to sit on the porch of an evening and listen to the **vespertine** serenade of insects."

Related word: **vespertide** (VES-pər-TĪD) noun.

vespine (VES-pīn)

From Latin *vespa,* meaning "a wasp."

An adjective worth brief examination even though it is not related to the word **vespertine.** Wasps, you see, are known for their habit of retiring before evening falls.

of or pertaining to a wasp or wasps.

"The wasp under discussion is none other than the universally feared **vespine** insect that forever threatens to scatter frightened picnickers."

Related word: **vespiary** (VES-pee-ER-ee) *noun.*

vestigial (ve-STIJ-ee-əl)

From Latin *vestigium,* meaning "footprint, footstep; trace, vestige."

of the nature of a vestige; surviving in a degenerate form.

"Traces of a **vestigial** tail were still perfectly visible in the first well-preserved specimen he was able to examine."

Related words: **vestige** (VES-tij) *noun;* **vestigially** (ves-TIJ-ee-ə-lee) *adverb.*

vicarious (vī-KAIR-ee-əs)

From Latin *vicarius*, meaning "substituting or substituted"; from *vicis*, meaning "a change, a turn; an office."

1. experienced imaginatively through another person.

"They convinced themselves that the **vicarious** thrill they felt for the honors bestowed on their son more than made up for all the years of self-denial they had gone through."

2. endured or substituted by one person in place of another.

"Ten men received **vicarious** punishment for the crimes of the actual saboteur."

Related words: **vicar** (VIK-ər) and **vicariate** (vī-KAIR-ee-it) *both nouns*; **vicariously** (vī-KAIR-ee-əs-lee) *adverb*; **vicariousness** (vī-KAIR-ee-əs-nis) noun; **vicarly** (VIK-ər-lee) *adjective*.

vicinal (VIS-ə-nl)

From Latin *vicinalis*, meaning "neighboring"; from *vicinitas*, meaning "neighborhood, nearness."

neighboring, adjacent; belonging to neighbors or a neighborhood.

"What they had not reckoned on was that the path going by their home would become **vicinal** rather than remain under their private ownership and so could be used by anyone who wanted to walk there."

Related words: **vicinity** (vi-SIN-i-tee) and **vicinage** (VIS-ə-nij) *both nouns*.

vincible (VIN-sə-bəl)

From Latin *vincibilis*, meaning "easily won"; from *vincere*, meaning "to conquer, subdue; overcome."

One of those English words much more commonly known by their negatives, in this case becoming **invincible,** with **in-,** meaning "not," added. We like to think of our side, our team, our army, our country as being invincible. Who wants to be associated with a **vincible** team?

conquerable, surmountable; susceptible to defeat or overthrow.

"From the very beginning of hostilities, Germany mistakenly regarded England as easily **vincible** in an air or ground war."

Related words: **vincibleness** (VIN-sə-bəl-nis) and **vincibility** (VIN-sə-BIL-i-tee) *both nouns*; **vincibly** (VIN-sə-blee) *adverb*.

vindictive (vin-DIK-tiv)

From Latin *vindicta,* meaning "revenge, vengeance."

1. of persons: given to gaining revenge; disposed to seek revenge.

"Our team, not realizing how **vindictive** our opponents could be, thought we were engaged in a sportsmanlike rivalry."

2. of actions, etc.: characterized by a desire for revenge.

"What they showed instead was a **vindictive** propensity that was certain to keep alive the bad feelings that lay at the core of our feud."

Related words: **vindictively** (vin-DIK-tiv-lee) *adverb;* **vindictiveness** (vin-DIK-tiv-nis) *noun;* **vindicatory** (VIN-di-kə-TOR-ee) and **vindicative** (vin-DIK-ə-tiv) *both adjectives* meaning "retributive."

virid. *See* **viridescent.**

viridescent (VIR-i-DES-ənt)

From Late Latin infinitive *viridescere,* meaning "to become green"; from Latin *viridis,* meaning "green; fresh, young, youthful."

greenish; slightly green or **virid.**

Virid (VIR-id) means green or verdant.

"Spring's **viridescent** landscapes lift one's spirits after the gray days of winter are past."

Related words: **viridescence** (VIR-i-DES-əns) and **viridity** (və-RID-i-tee) *both nouns.*

virulent (VIR-yə-lənt)

From Latin *virulentus,* meaning "poisonous"; from Latin *virus,* meaning "slime; poison; offensive smell."

This association with *virus* may explain why hapless physicians of an earlier time would stubbornly refuse to admit their ignorance, instead blaming everything unknown on a virus.

1. of disease: characterized by extreme malignancy or violence.

"He was not surprised to find that the **virulent** disease he had never seen before in temperate zones was common and usually fatal in the tropics."

2. of speech or writing: violently bitter; full of acrimony.

"He encountered **virulent** diatribes from his opponents when he first proposed careful examination of all available information on public housing."

3. of persons: full of hostility or enmity.

"She found it shocking to hear how bitterly **virulent** her candidate had become since being defeated for reelection."

Related words: **virulently** (VIR-yə-lənt-lee) *adverb*; **virulence** (VIR-yə-ləns) and **virulency** (VIR-yə-lən-see) *both nouns.*

vituperative (vī-TOO-pər-ə-tiv)
From English infinitive **vituperate**, meaning "to revile, vilify, berate"; from Latin infinitive *vituperare*, meaning "to find fault with."

1. of language: opprobrious; abusive, intemperate.

"The unexpected stream of **vituperative** condemnation he heaped on me made my ears burn."

2. of persons: given to abuse; employing abusive language.

"Our teacher would not put up with **vituperative** class monitors, no matter how talented they were otherwise."

Related words: **vituperatively** (vī-TOO-pər-ə-tiv-ly) *adverb*; **vituperation** (vī-TOO-pə-RAY-shən) *noun.*

votive (VOH-tiv)
From Latin *votivus*, meaning "promised in a vow; votive"; from *votum*, meaning "a longing" or "a vow."

offered in accordance with, or in consequence of, a vow.

"He did not know how he would be able to make a **votive** offering until he saw candles waiting nearby."

Related words: **vote** (voht) *verb* and *noun*; **votary** (VOH-tə-ree) *noun* and *adjective*; **votively** (VOH-tiv-lee) *adverb*; **votiveness** (VOH-tiv-nis) *noun.*

voyeuristic (VWAH-yə-RIS-tik)
From French *voyeur*, meaning "peeping Tom," with no hint of pleasantry suggested.

Rather, the implication is that of obtaining sexual gratification by stealing looks at sexually appealing objects or acts.

It must be noted that there is a mistaken but ever-increasing tendency to pronounce **voyeuristic** and related words as though the opening syllable sounded like the *voy* in *voyage*. Abandon this practice.

characteristic of peeping Toms, or **voyeurs** (vwah-YURZ).

"An excellent way of discouraging **voyeuristic** neighbors is to pull down all your shades."

Related words: **voyeurism** (vwah-YUR-iz-əm) *noun*; **voyeuristically** (VWAH-yə-RIS-tik-ə-lee) *adverb*.

vulpine (VUL-pīn)

From Latin *vulpinus*, meaning "cunning, crafty"; from *vulpes*, meaning "a fox."

Also given as **vulpecular** (vul-PEK-yə-lər).

crafty, cunning; resembling a fox.

"He was told his **vulpine** appearance puts people on guard instead of putting them at ease in his presence."

W

waggish (WAG-ish)

From Old Norse *vaga*, meaning "to sway"; from English **wag**, meaning "mischievous lad; habitual joker."

jocular; roguish, full of merriment; befitting a wag.

"My friends mistakenly thought of me as **waggish**, not realizing that beneath my jocund exterior lay brooding self-doubt."

Related words: **waggishly** (WAG-ish-lee) *adverb*; **waggishness** (WAG-ish-nis) and **waggery** (WAG-ə-ree) *both nouns.*

wanton (WON-tn)

From Middle English *wantowen*, literally meaning "ill-trained, undisciplined"; past participle of Old English infinitive *téon*, meaning "to train, discipline."

1. rebellious, undisciplined, without provocation; of children: naughty.

"The child's **wanton** disregard of others was the product of a complete lack of restraint practiced by his doting parents."

2. lascivious; lewd, unchaste; also, given to amorous adventures.

"It took just a few drinks to transform our shy drinking companion into a **wanton** satyr in perpetual pursuit of women."

3. excessively luxurious or extravagant.

"The **wanton** ways the young man had adopted soon exhausted his inheritance."

Related words: **wantonly** (WON-tn-lee) *adverb*; **wantonness** (WON-tn-nis) *noun.*

waspish (WOS-pish)

From English **wasp**, the familiar insect, as well as "a petulant person." Sometimes given as **waspy** (WOS-pee).

irascible; petulantly spiteful; snappish, quick to resent a small affront.

"Anybody is apt to be **waspish** if you try to speak with him before he's had his morning coffee."

Related words: **waspishly** (WOS-pish-lee) *adverb*; **waspishness** (WOS-pish-nis) *noun*.

well-knit (WEL-NIT)

From English verb **knit** + adverb **well**. Also given as **well-knitted**.

of a person's frame: firm, strong, and compactly built.

"The members of the wrestling team, with their **well-knit**, sturdy young bodies, were on their way to winning their third consecutive wrestling championship."

well-oiled (WEL-OILD)

From past participle of English verb **oil** + adverb **well**.

Anyone familiar with machinery knows the usefulness of oil in lubricating many moving parts, just as anyone with the slightest familiarity with slang knows that after a certain number of drinks of alcoholic beverages the imbiber may be said to be oiled, in fact **well-oiled**. Intoxicated, that is.

operating efficiently; also, drunk.

"**Well-oiled** machinery is essential for efficient functioning of my car, even if I am completely ignorant of basic mechanical equipment."

whorish (HOR-ish)

From English **whore**, meaning "a prostitute," + **-ish**, an adjectival suffix; from Latin *carus*, meaning "dear."

meretricious, unchaste; having the characteristics of a whore.

"Compared with the innocent girls I knew in my youth, the appearance and demeanor of today's women make them seem **whorish**."

Related words: **whorishly** (HOR-ish-lee) *adverb*; **whorishness** (HOR-ish-nis) *noun*.

willful (WIL-fəl)

From Old English *wilful*, meaning "willing"; from Latin *velle*, meaning "to wish, be willing."

Sometimes also spelled **wilful,** which is general practice among the British.

obstinately self-filled; perverse, unreasonably headstrong.

"The young mother was at a loss to know how to cope with the demands and rebelliousness of her **willful** child."

Related words: **willfully** (WIL-fəl-ee) *adverb*; **willfulness** (WIL-fəl-nis) *noun.*

willowy (WIL-oh-ee)
From Middle English *wilwe,* meaning "a willow."

of a person: lithe, tall and slender; resembling a willow in its gracefulness.

"Lisa was **willowy** and elegant, making the other, quite presentable girls in dancing class seem ungainly."

winsome (WIN-səm)
From Old English *wynsum* and Middle English *winsom,* both meaning "joyous."

comely; attractive in appearance, handsome; of winning character.

"Patricia was a **winsome** woman who made friends easily."

Related words: **winsomely** (WIN-səm-lee) *adverb*; **winsomeness** (WIN-səm-nis) *noun.*

witless (WIT-lis)
From Old English *witleas,* meaning "lacking wisdom."

stupid; lacking wit or intelligence; also, colloquially, extremely frightened.

"He had been scared **witless** at the idea of taking a test that might determine his entire future."

Related words: **witlessly** (WIT-lis-lee) *adverb*; **witlessness** (WIT-lis-nis) *noun.*

wizened (WIZ-ənd)
From Middle English infinitive *wisenen,* meaning "to wither."

of persons: shrunken and dried up; withered, shriveled.

"I was dismayed to find out that debilitating sickness had left my vigorous grandfather a **wizened** old man."

Related word: **wizen** (WIZ-ən) *verb.*

wonted (WAWN-tid)

From English noun **wont,** meaning "custom, habit," + **-ed,** an adjectival suffix forming a past participle, together meaning "accustomed."

accustomed, habituated; customary, habitual.

"My grandson Sam's **wonted** routine when he came to our house was first to peruse his favorite picture and then go around the rooms to inspect the other objects of special interest to him."

Related words: **wont** (wawnt) *verb;* **wontedly** (WAWN-tid-lee) *adverb;* **wontedness** (WAWN-tid-nis) *noun.*

wrongheaded (RAWNG-HED-id)

From English adjective **wrong,** meaning "incorrect," + **headed,** past participle of verb "head." Also given as **wrong-headed.**

stubborn; perversely or obstinately incorrect.

"We finally had to stop discussing politics because we always disagreed strongly and accused each other of being hopelessly **wrongheaded.**"

Related words: **wrongheadedly** (RAWNG-HED-id-lee) *adverb;* **wrongheadedness** (RAWNG-HED-id-nis) *noun.*

X

xenomorphic (ZEN-ə-MOR-fik)

From English **xeno-**, a combining form meaning "alien, strange"; from Greek *xénos*, a combining form meaning "a stranger, guest, alien, foreigner." The word is completed by English **-morphic,** from **-morphous,** a combining form meaning "having the shape or form of."

in an unusual form; formed differently than the normal.

"It was not until the very end of the expedition that they came upon strata yielding the predicted **xenomorphic** rock specimens."

Related word: **xenomorphically** (ZEN-ə-MOR-phi-kə-lee) *adverb.*

xenophilic (ZEN-ə-FIL-ik)

From English **xenophilia,** meaning "love of foreign people or things"; from Greek *xénos*, a combining form meaning "a stranger, guest," + Greek *-philos*, a combining form meaning "dear, beloved."

Also given as **xenophilous** (zen-O-fə-ləs).

fond of or attracted by foreign people or things.

"The **xenophilic** home lives of students usually can account for their subsequent careers as specialists in foreign language studies."

Related words: **xenophile** (ZEN-ə-FIL) and **xenophilia** (ZEN-ə-FIL-ee-ə) *both nouns.*

xenophobic (ZEN-ə-FOH-bik)

From English **xenophobia,** meaning "fear of foreign people or things"; from Greek *xénos*, a combining form meaning "a stranger, guest," + *-phobos*, a combining form meaning "afraid, panicked."

unreasonably fearful of foreign people or things.

"We never brought exchange students home when our father was there for fear that he would embarrass them and us with his **xenophobic** opinions."

Related words: **xenophobe** (ZEN-ə-FOHB) and **xenophobia** (ZEN-ə-FOH-bee-ə) *both nouns.*

xerophilous (zi-ROF-ə-ləs)

From English **xero-**, a combining form meaning "dry," + **-philous**, a combining form meaning "having an affinity for."

said especially of plants: adapted to living in hot, dry regions.

"A southern window in my dry, overheated apartment is hospitable to cacti and other **xerophilous** plants in my collection."

Related word: **xerophily** (zi-ROF-ə-lee) *noun.*

xerothermic (ZEER-ə-THUR-mik)

From English **xero-**, a combining form meaning "dry," + **-thermic,** a combining form meaning "heat or hot." In Greek *xerós* means "dry" and *thermós* means "hot."

adapted to an environment that is dry and hot.

"Our air-conditioned Greyhound was so comfortable that we could scarcely appreciate what our guide was telling us about the **xerothermic** environment outside our bus."

xylophagous (zī-LOF-ə-gəs)

From Greek *xylophágos,* from *xylo-*, a combining form meaning "wood," + *-phagous*, a combining form meaning "eating, feeding on."

eating wood; destroying lumber.

"The first sign of the nightmare of **xylophagous** infestation of our library was a small pile of sawdust on the floor of the main reading room."

Related word: **xylophage** (ZĪ-lə-FAYJ) *noun.*

Y

yearling (YEER-ling)
From Dutch *jaerlingh* and German *Jährling*, nouns meaning "an animal in its second year of life."

of an animal: being a year old; in its second year.

"All entries for two of the day's races were identified as **yearling** maiden ponies."

yeasty (YEE-stee)
From English **yeast**, a leavening agent, + -y, a suffix meaning "inclined to."

ebullient; frothy, exuberant; youthful, given to excitement, agitation, change, etc.; light and superficial.

"Her senior year, when she was editor of the school's literary magazine, was a **yeasty** period for her."

Related words: **yeastily** (YEE-sti-lee) *adverb*; **yeastiness** (YEE-stinis) *noun*.

youngblood (YUNG-BLUD)
From English **young** + **blood**, combinations with such meanings as "vigor, youth, and youthful persons."

having the vigor of youthful persons, new ideas, etc.

"The company's personnel department had finally become interested in making **youngblood** additions to our aging sales force."

Z

zaftig (ZAHF-tik)

From Yiddish *zaftik*, meaning "juicy, succulent"; from German *saftig*, meaning "juicy." Also given as **zoftig** (ZAHF-tik).

of a woman: sexy; plump; well-proportioned, curvaceous.

"There was no doubt he was interested only in **zaftig** females, whose overflowing ripeness would prove a fitting complement for his own carefully tended masculinity."

zealous (ZEL-əs)

From Latin *zelus*, from Greek *zàlos*, meaning "zeal."

devoted; intensely earnest, actively enthusiastic; eagerly desirous.

"After he heard his first Louis Armstrong recording he became a **zealous** jazz fan and started his extensive record collection."

Related words: **zealously** (ZEL-əs-lee) *adverb*; **zealousness** (ZEL-əs-nis) *noun*.

zymotic (zī-MOT-ik)

From Greek *zymotikós*, meaning "cause fermentation."

caused by or as if by a process resembling fermentation; pertaining to a process akin to this.

"The pubs in her neighborhod were closed down by an inspector who mistakenly believed the beer served there was afflicted with a **zymotic** disease."

Related words: **zymosis** (zī-MOH-sis) *noun*; **zymotically** (zī-MOT-ik-ə-lee) *adverb*.